KT-487-111

CEREBRAL PALSIED
CHILD AT HOME

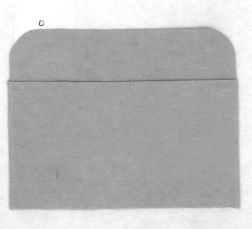

The first edition of this book was approved by the
CHARTERED SOCIETY OF PHYSIOTHERAPY
for the award of a
FELLOWSHIP
to the author.

HANDLING THE YOUNG CEREBRAL PALSIED CHILD AT HOME

BY

NANCIE R. FINNIE. F.C.S.P.

Superintendent Physiotherapist, Department of Paediatrics,
Charing Cross Hospital, London.

with contributions by

Dr Jack Bavin, M.B., B.S., B.Sc., F.R.C. Psych., D.P.M.
Helen Mueller, Speech Therapist
Mary Gardner, B.Sc.(Econ)., Dip.Ed., Dip.Psych.

Sketches by
Margaret Inkpen, O.T.R.

Assistant Supervisor, Occupational Therapy,
The Glenrose Hospital, Edmonton, Canada.

SECOND EDITION

WILLIAM HEINEMANN MEDICAL BOOKS LTD
LONDON

First published 1968
Reprinted 1969
Reprinted 1971

Second Edition 1974
Reprinted 1976
Reprinted 1978
Reprinted 1981
Reprinted 1984

© Nancie R. Finnie, F.C.S.P. 1974

I.S.B.N. 0 433 10381 7

Photoset by Seventy Set Ltd, London

Printed in Great Britain by
Biddles Ltd, Guildford, Surrey

This book is dedicated to
Berta Bobath

CONTRIBUTORS

'Parents Problems'
by Dr. Jack Bavin, MB, BS, B.Sc., F.R.C.Psych., D.P.M.

'Feeding' by Helen Mueller   *Speech Therapist*

'Speech' by Helen Mueller   *Speech Therapist*

'The Psychologist and the Child with Cerebral Palsy'
by Mary Gardner, B.Sc. (Econ.), Dip. Ed., Dip. Psych.

CONTENTS

PREFACE BY HUGH JOLLY, M.A., M.D., F.R.C.P., D.C.H.
Consultant Paediatrician   ix

FOREWORD BY DR. K. BOBATH, M.D., D.P.M.
AND MRS. B. BOBATH, F.C.S.P., S.A.A.O.T. (Hon.)   x

Chapter

1 GENERAL GUIDANCE   1

2 PARENTS' PROBLEMS   12

3 MOVEMENT   32

4 BASIC PRINCIPLES OF HANDLING   51

5 SLEEPING   68

6 TOILET TRAINING   75

7 BATHING   82

8 DRESSING   90

9 FEEDING   111

10 SPEECH   131

11 CARRYING   139

12 PRAMS, PUSH-CHAIRS AND CHAIRS   151

13 HAMMOCKS, WEDGES AND PRONE BOARDS   179

14 AIDS TO MOBILITY   191

15 THE PSYCHOLOGIST AND THE CHILD WITH
     CEREBRAL PALSY   200

16 THE FUNDAMENTALS OF GRASP AND
     MANIPULATION   211

17 PLAY   226

APPENDIX I   *Early Stages of Normal Development*   266

APPENDIX II   *Questionnaire*   275

GLOSSARY   287

SUPPLIERS OF EQUIPMENT AND ACCESSORIES   290

INDEX   301

PREFACE TO THE SECOND EDITION

This is a book for the parents of children with cerebral palsy. Its message, however, is so important that it should be read by all those caring for such children, including doctors, therapists, teachers and nurses. An American paediatrician, while telling me how valuable he found the first edition, had the title as his only criticism, feeling that this should indicate more clearly the value of the book for doctors and therapists. While agreeing with this comment I think that Miss Finnie is wise to have stressed the importance of handling by parents since this is often overlooked.

Miss Finnie emphasizes the vital role of parents in the day to day handling of their child and the need for them to be taught this skill. This is additional to treatment from therapists. Parents, as the most important members of the team caring for the handicapped child, must be deeply involved from the start. This start should be as early as possible, preferably while the child is still a baby, so that physiotherapy can have its maximum influence.

The management of the child with cerebral palsy involves handling, treatment and play all of which must be organised through the parents. No child should be treated in isolation.

The enormous success of the first edition, in terms of copies sold and translations made, speaks for itself. There never has been a book for parents quite like it. Its success lies in the skill, experience and understanding of Nancie Finnie who has helped countless cerebral palsied children and their parents to a happier and fuller life. It is the outcome of many years working with Dr. and Mrs. Bobath in the Western Cerebral Palsy Centre and now of working in the Child Development Centre of Charing Cross Hospital. The changes in the new edition reflect the modern multidisciplinary approach to the problem. The value of this edition is enhanced by the contributions of Dr. Jack Bavin, Mrs. Mary Gardner and Miss Helen Mueller as well as by the artistry and skill of Miss Margaret Inkpen.

HUGH JOLLY
MA., MD., FRCP, DCH

Charing Cross Hospital, London,
January 1974

FOREWORD TO THE FIRST EDITION

A normal newborn baby is helpless and totally dependent. He is unable to raise and hold up his head, to sit up or to maintain any position against the pull of gravity. He cannot by himself control any position such as sitting or kneeling and without support would fall. His head wobbles and he cannot hold it firmly in one position by himself. Gradually, as the brain matures, he begins to control positions against gravity. For instance, when the baby is about 5 to 6 weeks old and is placed on his tummy he will raise his head quite well, and from then onwards the control of his head will improve until, at about 6 months, he can raise it high and look around. From the 5th month onwards the baby can lift his head when lying on his back. Watch yourself when trying to stand up from lying on your tummy – the first thing you will do is raise your head and then put your arms down to push yourself up, from this you will see how important head control is in order to stand up. During the day-time all people hold their heads properly in line with the neck and the body, it is held there firmly controlled and can be moved and turned freely, and the eyes can look into the surrounding space or at a book, carefully following a line. Head control is, therefore, one of the most important factors of human development in the physical and the mental field.

Another important factor of child development is the ability, starting at about 6 months, to extend and use his extended arms for support. We use our arms for pushing ourselves up to sitting, for getting into a kneeling position in readiness for standing up. Even as adults we use the support of our arms if for some reason we have to get onto our hands and knees, or to get in and out of the bath. We also need the protective extension of our arms, if, when sitting or standing someone pushes us and we lose our balance. This shows that head control and the ability to use extended arms for support are fundamental patterns of normal movements against gravity and for balance, and develop in all of us very early in life, however, an adult person will only need the use of his arms and hands occasionally for support.

In normal circumstances the muscles of the body work in such a way that we are able to maintain balance in all activities, freeing the use of our arms for many and varied activities and skills, and only rarely for the maintenance of our postures.

What goes wrong with the child with cerebral palsy?

Due to damage to the brain in earliest childhood, the development of a cerebral palsied child is retarded, or stopped, and becomes disorganised and abnormal. In many children with cerebral palsy, therefore, one sees insufficient, or a total lack of, head control, and also an incompletely developed ability to use the arms and hands for support, for reaching out, for grasp and for manipulation, the child also lacks balance and control of his postures, especially in sitting, standing and walking.

The spastic child is stiff, if he is on his back it will be seen that his head is usually pulled back and he cannot raise it, or does so only with great effort. Usually, he is unable to bring his shoulders and arms forward and therefore he cannot bend his spine nor sit up nor pull himself to sitting. If you pull him up to sitting, his head falls or pushes back, he cannot turn over as his shoulders are pulling back, when he sits his head is not straight – it either pulls back or slumps forward. He cannot extend his arms for support and falls backwards or sideways, even if he has fairly good head control and can extend his arms, he cannot bend his spine and hips and has to use his arms for support. Watch him lying on his tummy, if he is totally involved he will not be able to raise his head or to push himself up with his arms, he is therefore unable to get himself to kneeling and from there to sitting.

If a child is only partially involved, if for instance only the legs are affected, he may be able to sit up by bringing his head forward and by pulling himself up to sitting with his arms, but he will have to use his arms for support and if he lifts them to reach out for an object he may lose his balance and fall backwards or sideways. Fundamentally, therefore, the motor difficulties of children with cerebral palsy may be regarded as the result of brain damage which interferes with the normal ability to move and maintain posture and balance.

The treatment and management of children suffering from cerebral palsy requires the combined effort of doctors, therapists and parents.

It has long been felt that if the child is to make progress the parents have to play an active and intelligent part in the total treatment programme. This applies especially to a baby or young child who spends most of the time with his mother. Home management, that is, the way the mother handles her child when playing with him, when carrying, feeding, dressing, bathing and potting him, can mean a great deal in furthering or hindering a child's progress. The mother should not be left without detailed advice and guidance because this has often proved an obstacle to successful treatment.

A great deal of time should be spent on teaching the parent how to handle her child at home to the best advantage, so that any improvement made during treatment can be carried over, used and reinforced at home. Though advice and guidance is most important, the mother should not just be taught what to do and how to do it, but must learn to understand why she should do certain things, and why she should not do others.

In short, she must understand her child, his difficulties and the things he might be able to do if helped in the right way at any stage of his treatment and development. She also needs to know something about normal child development, its importance for learning new activities and in what way damage to the brain has slowed down her child's development or caused it to be abnormal.

This book should be of help to therapists as well as to parents and teachers. It is the result of Miss Finnie's special interest and great experience in dealing with these problems for thirteen years as Deputy Principal of the Western Cerebral Palsy Centre, London. No child with cerebral palsy is like another and general advice that might apply to all children is not of much use. Miss Finnie has attempted to give specific advice on the difficulties and the handling of various types of children. She says, 'if your child is like this . . . . then you do that . . . .'. This way of tackling the problem has not been attempted before, and it is this, together with the many illustrations, which makes the book so valuable to parents, teachers and all those caring for these children.

DR. K. BOBATH
MRS. B. BOBATH

ACKNOWLEDGEMENTS

I thank Mrs. Berta Bobath and her husband Dr. Karl Bobath, the originators of the Neuro-Developmental Treatment for cerebral palsy for their personal interest and the invaluable experience of working with them for many years at the Western Cerebral Palsy Centre, London. I thank Dr. Hugh Jolly Consultant Paediatrician, Charing Cross Hospital, who has kindly written the Preface to this second edition.

The acceptance in the U.K. and in so many other countries of the edition first published in 1968 and the friendly prompting of my colleagues, for which I thank them, has encouraged me to write this second edition, its scope has been extended and strengthened by the contributions of Dr. Jack Bavin, Mrs. Mary Gardner and Miss Helen Mueller.

I am indebted to Frances Hall for her continued interest and to Pamela Knowles and Elizabeth Blyth who have so patiently and skilfully typed and re-typed the manuscript and for the advice, help and encouragement of my colleagues in The Child Development Centre of Charing Cross Hospital and to my husband for his patience and help throughout the preparation of this second edition.

Sketches
Miss Inkpen qualified as an Occupational Therapist in 1961. After four years work in England, two and a half years were spent at The Glenrose School Hospital, Edmonton, Alberta, Canada. Returning to England in 1968 she took the Bobath Course at The Western Cerebral Palsy Centre, London, and until 1970 worked at The Cerebral Palsy Unit, Harperbury Hospital, Herts. She is now engaged as Assistant Supervisor of Occupational Therapy at The Glenrose School Hospital where she also holds the position of Co-ordinator of the Nursery Programme for handicapped pre-school children. Miss Inkpen has combined her skill as an artist in this field with her wide qualifications and experience as an Occupational Therapist to produce the series of drawings which do so much to illuminate the text.

Chapter 1

GENERAL GUIDANCE

Treating and handling a child suffering from cerebral palsy involves tackling a wide range of problems. In this work the co-operation of the parents is vital, for only when parents and therapists work together as a team can a child be given the best opportunities for developing his capabilities, however limited they may be. Many years of experience in treating children with cerebral palsy has proved this to be true. It is a mistake for parents to think that, having handed over their child to experts, their responsibilities, so far as handling and treatment are concerned, are lessened, nothing could be further from the truth; rather it should mark the beginning of a partnership between parent and therapist in the overall care and treatment of the child.

This book deals mainly with the baby and the child up to five years of age – the period during which a child is handled and taught mainly by his parents. It will be confined to the difficulties most commonly met with, setting out in some detail the causes of the difficulties, and giving advice on how to deal with the problems. *Not all the difficulties described will necessarily apply to any one child.* Children with cerebral palsy may be spastic, athetoid, ataxic or flaccid (floppy) and their intelligence may range from normal to subnormal. There may also be associated handicaps affecting vision, hearing and speech, specific learning problems and possibly some physical deformity or emotional involvement.

All these aspects have to be taken into account when assessing the problems of each child. Furthermore, in many cases, the chronological age of the child does not correspond with his developmental age; sometimes this can be at a generally lower level in all aspects of development, at other times there is a 'scatter' in achievements. A child of four, for example, may not have progressed as far as his movements and skills are concerned beyond the stage of that of a young baby, while another child may be within normal limits, as regards gross motor skills, but be unable to speak.

When considering the examples and suggestions given in this book it must always be remembered that not all children will be affected exactly in the manner described and that parents will need to adapt the advice given to the needs of their child.

Many children, for example, will be able to control the position of the head and to use their hands quite well, while others will find it difficult or impossible. There are some children who although able to manipulate

1

a toy or object are unable to understand their use. Some children, when lying on their backs, may have stiff legs but fairly good use of their arms and body and can therefore move away from this position, while others when on their backs may also press their heads and shoulders back onto the support, unable to use their arms and hands and are therefore helpless. While the majority of severely handicapped children may find it difficult to raise their heads when lying on their tummies, there will be a few who will find it impossible to put their heads down onto the floor or support.

It is also realised that the abilities of parents will vary and that some will find the suggestions difficult to carry out or to adapt. Even so, it is hoped that the advice will not be discarded too readily, but that every attempt will be made to relate it to their own abilities and to those of the child.

It is understandable that having purchased a book on a subject of interest to parents, that you will be inclined either to skim through the text and concentrate on the sketches and captions, or, to read it straight through from beginning to end.

When you have read the first three chapters, I suggest that you study the 'Questionnaire' carefully and apply the questions to your child, and discuss your findings with all those who help you to look after him. If your child is under a year old also read 'Early Stages of Normal Development'. A knowledge of *normal* development in its early phases helps us to understand how each stage of development prepares for and overlaps the next. By looking briefly at the important stages in the motor development of a *normal* baby at the same time considering his development in vision, hearing and speech, we see how they progress along the same broad lines.

The early emotional and social aspects of development are covered in the chapters by Dr. Bavin and Mary Gardner.

A study of the stages of early development also helps us to assess what degree of departure from the *normal* is suffered by the cerebral palsied child. We emphasise that the therapist when planning a programme of treatment, whilst having due regard for this knowledge, takes fully into account the pathology of the child which is the result of the damage to his brain.

Remember that, to some extent, this book can be used as a work of reference, and with the growing knowledge and understanding of your child's problems you will be able with the guidance of your therapist to work out additional ways in which you can help him.

Make a point of learning about the many additional products that become available from time to time, as often with minor adaptations they will prove most useful.

The essential purpose of this book is to enlist the co-operation of parents and to suggest ways of handling the child at home. *It must be emphasised that, although good handling at home is an important and essential adjunct to treatment, it cannot take the place of treatment and must not be regarded as a substitute.*

I cannot emphasise too strongly that this book is *not* a treatment manual, it is, as the title suggests, for use in the *home management* of the cerebral palsied child by the parents. Please look upon the advice given as only *complementary* to treatment, and encourage your child to use, during all his waking hours, the new abilities that he acquires during treatment sessions.

Do not be tempted to spur your child on to achievements that are beyond his capacity and do disregard casual suggestions made to you as to the home management of your child until you have discussed them with your therapists.

The First Interview

The first meeting between the parents and the therapist will be concerned with finding out what the parents feel are the main problems of the child, assessing his abilities and disabilities and with the older child how much independence he has achieved, and then planning treatment and home management for the immediate future. The therapist will explain step by step what she is going to do and why, and what she hopes to achieve, stage by stage, from treatment. She will stress the importance of careful handling by the parents during the child's first years, and particularly during the critical first year, for at no other time does a child develop so rapidly as during the first twelve months. Indeed, it is impossible to over-emphasise the value of early treatment in combination with good handling, for the earlier the treatment and the younger the child, the less the degree of probable abnormality. If we disregard abnormalities that are *not* due to cerebral palsy, contractures and deformities are not usually present in the baby who may have cerebral palsy.

Any incipient abnormality which may exist in the very young child will obviously respond better to early treatment than to later treatment, when the abnormal condition may have become more established. Recognising the importance of early treatment, it will be clear that the correct handling of the baby by his parents, in support of treatment, is of equal importance.

As the aim in all treatment is to get improvement in functional activities, the therapist will explain to the parents that treatment should not be regarded as a separate half-hour session each day, but that it should be directly related to the activities of the day. This is why the co-operation of the parents is so important – so much can be done at home that is not possible in a treatment room.

The following examples help to illustrate the point. During treatment, a child may begin to acquire balance in sitting and start to reach out and hold on to a support, that is to say he has developed good head and trunk control and the ability to grasp with extended arms. When the

3

child has acquired these new abilities in treatment you should immediately ask yourself such questions as, is he being given too much support when carried, is he being supported unnecessarily when sitting on his pot, are we continuing to feed him when in fact he is able to grasp a spoon and is ready to start to feed himself and so on? His new ability to balance and grasp has made a number of new skills possible, and opportunities to use these skills will come throughout the day and no time should be wasted before encouraging him to further achievements. An older child, may be able to sit well learning how to grasp and pull, and grasp and push, and he should be encouraged to make use of this new ability when, for example, pulling his socks on and off and when dressing and undressing, and by helping you with any activity in the home that incorporates the movements he has learned.

Approach to Treatment

The first step towards effective handling and treatment calls for a full understanding of the child's abilities and disabilities, accordingly, we strongly advise that, whenever possible, the mother as well as the father should together attend the early sessions with the therapists. If, from the beginning, the basic problems are fully understood, the advice will be meaningful and future re-assessment and changes in the child's programme of treatment and handling will be easier to understand and to carry out.

The early sessions with the therapists will also give the parents an opportunity to discuss the main problems as they see them. If, as we sometimes find, there is a difference of opinion or attitude between the parents concerning the child's general behaviour, emotional difficulties, problems or achievements, the time to discuss them is during these early sessions.

As Mary Gardner has pointed out in her chapter, never be overawed by experts. If you cannot understand the reasons why certain handling or treatment techniques have been suggested, do not hesitate to ask for an explanation as in doing so, not only will you be helping yourself and your child but just as importantly your therapist. Ask for further explanations if, for example, you are not clear as to the reasons *why* your child finds a certain movement difficult or impossible, or you are not sure exactly how much of a movement he can do by himself and *when* and *where* you should give help, and even more important when to withdraw your support entirely.

Sometimes your therapist may use a medical or technical term that worries you because you do not understand, do not worry, as all you have to do is ask for an explanation.

It is possible that you will find, to begin with, that the speed of handling that you have been asked to apply to get a desired reaction, or a certain grip or hold that you have been asked to do, or even the aims behind certain exercises are not clear to you. If any of these points apply

4

to you, discuss them immediately with your therapists, try to demonstrate your problems and together you can work out a solution. Do not give up, perhaps feeling that it is technically too difficult for you.

If you have found, as so often is the case, a new way of handling, or an idea for treatment that enables both you and the child to achieve more, tell your therapist. We are always learning from parents and often get useful suggestions that we pass on to other parents.

Approach to handling in functional activities

The cerebral palsied child is not only limited to movements which are stereotyped, but is also limited in his reactions and responses to being moved. If your child is severely affected he will be almost helpless when you handle, bath, feed and dress him, and be unable to move or adjust himself to any changes in movement. The spastic child will be stiff, and become stiffer if not handled well as you move him; he cannot move sufficiently to balance, which makes him insecure and tense. The athetoid child, because of his involuntary movements and the constantly changing tone of his muscles, easily loses his balance and falls over.

When you start to teach your child to feed, dress or wash himself, it is important to realise that a *normal* child needs assistance in these activities for some years before he can do them by himself. Consider how the *normal* child reacts when you bath, dress, feed, carry him and so on. He moves with you rather than against you, it is easy to lift his arms up to wash or dress him, his hands are not tightly fisted – they open easily. If you put anything over his head – his jersey or shirt, for example, he automatically pushes his head through, if you part his legs to put on his nappy he offers no resistance as you move him. When you pick him up he holds up his head, if he feels insecure he can immediately grasp and hold on to you. His natural self protective reactions and his ability to balance enable him to adjust and change his posture if he is uncomfortable while being handled. For example, most children dislike having their noses and ears cleaned and will move and dodge in the hope of avoiding this attention – if this does not have the desired effect they use their hands to push mother away.

The cerebral palsied child cannot do these things. All that he can do is to cry and become stiff and frightened. If he is the 'floppy' type of child he will have to be supported and held everywhere or he will fall. Because of this we must handle a cerebral palsied child slowly, and give him a chance to make his own adjustment as we move him, supporting him where and when necessary, but waiting and giving him time to do whatever he possibly can by himself.

It is most important, when anything is being done for the child, that he should not be passive, let him see what is being done and talk to him about it. Name the parts of his body, and describe his clothes and their colour as you dress him, and the movements he is making. For example say, 'help me to push your foot into your shoe', and 'lean forward so that

5

I can get your coat around your shoulders'.

By these means not only is the child being taught to understand language, but is learning something of the relationship of one part of his body to another, all designed to give him experiences of normal movement. This attitude should be applied to all everyday activities. A cerebral palsied child takes far longer than a *normal* child to understand and to store information, therefore constant repetition is of real value, it should always be borne in mind that he does not have the same opportunity as a *normal* child of learning by trial and error and by experimenting.

One should try at all times to enlist the child's co-operation. Within reasonable limits ask him what he would like to wear, what and how much he would like to eat. We all like to sit back and have things done for us, the more difficult a task, the greater our readiness to hand it over to someone else. How much more does this apply to the cerebral palsied child? He enjoys attention and becomes used to having everything done for him, parents quite naturally get used to doing everything for him and, in time, stop expecting any help from him.

Parents should keep a notebook to record new problems, achievements, and when necessary any specific exercises or notes on handling, or points on which they may need further explanation. These records are studied by the therapist at the beginning of each session and are of real help. When your child is young it is your observations in the home environment that are so important. If, for example, you think that physically your child is making progress but that his concentration span is short, that he moves around but aimlessly and does not seem inquisitive, do ask for help. It may be that his programme of handling and treatment needs to be reviewed, that more time should be spent on other aspects of his development and less on the physical side. It is pointless to continue with a planned programme if all-round progress is not being made, rather it is a time for re-assessment, to determine whether too much has been asked of the child, or over-emphasis is being applied in one area at the expense of another, or, in fact, that the child could be more independent if approached in a different way. It may be that he has lost interest as he is not receiving sufficient support and interest from his family to make any effort on his part worthwhile, or that he is not being allowed to make his own mistakes, in effect too much help is being given to him.

Some children have the additional handicap of delayed or specific speech difficulties, or of vision, hearing, and specific learning disabilities. It is not sufficient merely for you to *know* that these problems exist, but also to realise and understand how they affect the overall development of your child. The programme devised for your child will not be divided into so many minutes for movement, speech or general skills, but will be an integrated one covering all these aspects at the same time.

Time is precious, even more so when there are other children in the family, *but no cerebral palsied child will ever become independent unless he is*

6

given an opportunity to try. To compete is always stimulating so, whenever possible, let your child dress, wash and eat with the other children in the family, in this way he will be much more inclined to try to help himself.

Admittedly some children's handicaps make it impossible for them to do very much for themselves, but with correct help and guidance and the avoidance of excessive effort on the part of the child, he will learn to do more and more for himself. Avoid *excessive* effort, as failure can lead to tenseness and frustration with the probable result that the child will give up. Even if a child cannot use his hands or speak, he is sure to have some way of indicating what he wants and in this way he can co-operate, for example, if you are building a house with bricks, have a book with different pictures of houses and get him to act as 'foreman' and 'direct proceedings'. He can choose the type of house he wants you to build, decide on the type of roof, the number of windows, and where he wants the door to be, and so on. When the house has been built he will know that he has taken an active part in its construction.

Visual defects
Many children suffer the additional handicap of visual defects. They may have a squint, an inability to focus with one or both eyes, nystagmus (continual oscillation of the eyeballs) or other oculo-motor defects. Visual disorders call for specialised advice and treatment from an ophthalmologist. If glasses are prescribed you must see that they are worn.

Hearing defects
Some cerebral palsied children suffer from the additional handicap of deafness, or the partial handicap of being able to distinguish only certain qualities of pitch or tone, and in such cases a hearing aid may be prescribed by a specialist. As hearing disorders call for highly specialised treatment and advice, no attempt will be made to offer advice on such disorders.

If difficulties should arise, seek expert advice immediately; do not discard a hearing aid because your child cannot cope – it will take time and patience, sometimes a minor adjustment will solve the problems.

Speech
The delays and difficulties in acquiring the ability to speak, which so often add to the handicaps of cerebral palsied children, are dealt with by Miss Helen Mueller, a chapter which, I stress, will amply reward careful study by those parents whose children suffer from any speech defect.

Speech is a very complex skill. The muscles and organs used for it are secondary; the primary purpose of these organs is to enable us to breathe and feed. In fact a good 'speech pattern' is based on good feeding and breathing patterns.

Crying, babbling and cooing are forms of expression for a baby, indicating his discomfort, anger or pleasure. He tends to make noises

7

when he is happy and contented, especially when he is being nursed or at feeding times. It is therefore important that mealtimes should be times of enjoyment, for at this time the child has a very close emotional link with his mother. Often, after he has been fed and is happy and close to his mother and having used his lips and tongue in feeding, a baby starts playing with sounds – a preparation for speech. It is noticeable that if anything happens to disturb this close relationship the child tends to stop reacting in this way and may even cry. As he grows older, and mealtimes become more of a social occasion with the rest of the family, he expresses his satisfaction or dislike of his food, saying 'yes' or 'no' when offered food, he names the food and makes simple requests such as 'more', 'give me', and so on.

If a cerebral palsied child is to learn to speak, patience is essential. We must wait and listen, and give him a chance to try to speak and express himself at his own speed. If we are satisfied merely to interpret his nods and looks, why should the child be expected to make the effort, which is obviously called for, to speak, if he can get what he wants without trying to express himself? Again, the child should not be spoken to in baby language. By doing so we rob him of the opportunity to increase his vocabulary and to understand the meaning of words that he will need when eventually he starts to speak.

Listening is difficult for many cerebral palsied children, one reason being a lack of ability to concentrate, a point we sometimes overlook. The child not only needs to listen to the words we speak, but to the emphasis that we put on certain words, the variation in tone we use and so on. Try, if you can, to set aside a time each day when you speak and listen to your child alone, without the radio or television, this will give him a chance to attend to what you say and to interpret the meaning of your words. If you are playing with him and he makes a new sound, make him aware he has done so by showing him that you are pleased. Repeat the sound several times and then ask him to do it with you, helping him with his specific difficulties as your speech therapist advises. In this way you will reduce the effort needed and the difficulties the child so often has when he is asked to make a specific sound.

If he cannot speak, or can only say a few words with difficulty, he will be unable to ask the many questions which the *normal* child asks and will be deprived of the opportunity to learn by asking questions. You can help him by talking to him about the things you are doing. Give him a running commentary as you cook and do the housework, and while you dress or wash him, you yourself asking the questions and giving him the answers. Do this when you take him for a walk, or look out of the window, and describe to him what is going on.

When he starts to talk, encourage him to describe what he sees in the room. If he can walk or crawl, get him to name the objects he has passed, or, as he plays, to talk to you about his interests and what he is doing or plans to do. See if he can remember what you bought at the shops and what he saw when he was out for a walk – verbal contact is essential if sounds and speech are to be achieved; if he always remains in one room, or goes out for the same walk every day, his experiences of daily life will be very limited. These are a few suggestions which may help and encourage him to speak and to understand the world around him.

A stay in hospital

An occasion may arise when your child has to spend a period in hospital. A stay in hospital, especially for the first time, is sometimes a frightening experience for a child, and of course an anxious time for parents. Before your child goes into hospital, a visit by parents with him to meet the staff and see the ward will prove well worthwhile. For the older child, a great deal of anxiety and insecurity can, to some extent, be avoided if the reasons for his stay in hospital are explained to him.

Inevitably the unhappiness of parting will be hard for a child with cerebral palsy, as he will have spent most of his time with his mother, providing him with a complete sense of security by her proficient handling and her understanding of his problems and special needs, so do make sure that all those taking care of him in hospital are given full information regarding his handling.

A short explanation of his basic problems will be an immense aid to the staff and will help him to feel secure and to settle in quickly. If he is unable to speak and makes his needs known by gesture, explain how he lets you know when he needs you, that he is uncomfortable or that he wants to go to the toilet, or wants a drink of water, and how for example he indicates 'yes' or 'no'.

Feeding is often a problem and where difficulties in chewing, swallowing or drinking are present, information on how you cope will always be welcomed by the staff. If a special plate, cup or spoon is used bring them with him. If you have any special ways of dressing, potting or toileting your child, or he has problems at night, let the staff know. If he has a special chair or other equipment, not available in the ward, ask the ward sister whether she thinks you should bring it in. Be sure to bring his favourite toy with him; it is often a great comfort especially if the child's ability to use his hands is limited and information regarding the type of toys he enjoys is always welcomed.

If your child has to have an operation it is important, when he is old enough to understand, that he is told in a simple way the reasons for the operation, and has the procedure explained to him. If a plaster is to be put on after the operation, tell him why beforehand, as children naturally feel let down, if for example, they are told that the operation will help to make them walk and then they wake up and find their leg in plaster and that they have to stay in bed for another week.

If there are play specialists in the wards, they will, of course, in addition to helping the child settle down and cope with hospital life, also help to prepare the child for his operation, explaining the various

9

procedures in the form of a game. As through play the child will be able to express any fears or worries he may have about medical tests or operations.

You will find it worthwhile to read 'Paul in Hospital' by C. Jessel and H. Jolly, published by Methuen's Children's Books.

Toy Libraries Association

In some countries toy libraries are being set up for mentally and physically handicapped children. These libraries provide a very practical service for the child and his family. Sometimes they are run by professional people with a special interest in play, such as psychologists, teachers and therapists, others are run by the parents and volunteers. These libraries often combine a small reference library with various publications and catalogues dealing with play and toys. Through a newsletter and an up-to-date 'ABC Toy Index', the Association passes on guidance about the right toys and play to the individual toy libraries.

The advantages of using a toy library are two-fold. Firstly, it enables the child to have a variety of toys of particular value for developing special skills at different stages in his development, secondly, it enables parents to discuss the various learning situations possible with each toy. A toy library also provides an excellent opportunity for an exchange of ideas between parents and members of the library and parents with one another. If there is a toy library in your locality it is well worth a visit.

Swimming and Riding

I am often asked whether we would recommend these activities as being beneficial for cerebral palsied children. *Provided* they are carried out under qualified supervision, these sports serve a useful purpose in developing self confidence and a degree of independence, apart of course, from the pleasure they give the children.

Social Services

In addition to the medical services there are many organisations in this and in other countries which have been set up, either locally or at government level, to assist handicapped children and their families with literature, practical aid and financial assistance. The degree of assistance available obviously varies in different parts of the world and even in different areas in the United Kingdom. It is clearly impracticable in this book, which has been translated into many foreign languages, to provide details. The purpose however is served by reminding you that if you need help it is available and that you are entitled to it.

NOTE

Considerable publicity has recently been given to the highly inflammable nature of certain types of foam and similar materials. I therefore advise parents when buying these materials to make sure that they are fireproof, also to be sure when using foam materials that they are adequately covered to avoid the risk of injury resulting from the child getting pieces of foam into his mouth.

Chapter 2

PARENTS' PROBLEMS

By Jack Bavin

Dr. J.T.R. Bavin, M.B., B.S., B.Sc., F.R.C.Psych., D.P.M. Consultant Psychiatrist, Leavesden Hospital and Charing Cross Hospital.
Member of the Standing Mental Health Advisory Committee to the Department of Health and Social Security.

The Problem of Acceptance

No-one wants a handicapped child. We all want fit, handsome, intelligent children who will do well in the competitive society we live in, and 'be a credit to us'. We even have baby competitions to find the most beautiful baby. It is small wonder, therefore, that parents worry during the end of pregnancy about what sort of baby they are going to have, and become acutely distressed if they give birth to a damaged or imperfect child.

The parents' distress can be, and usually is, severe. At first the feelings of guilt, shame, despair, and self-pity may be overwhelming, so that only the agony of longing for a way out may be experienced. In some these feelings may even give way to a resolve to end the baby's and one's own life. If the distress of meeting the situation is intolerable there may be total rejection of the child, or denial that there is anything wrong with him, or a belief that he belongs to someone else.

Torturing questions flood the mind: "What did I do wrong? Why did it happen to me! What is wrong with me?" The answers are no less distressing: "Perhaps I can't produce *normal* children. I damaged its brain because my pelvis is small – they said it was. I wish I had never got married. How I hate the other mothers who have *normal* babies." And then, maybe more questions such as: "Oh, why am I thinking these terrible thoughts – what sort of person am I? He needs a mother to love him, and yet we were going to abandon him."

The initial turmoil may give way to sadness, a feeling of desolation and isolation, and a longing for the lost, *normal* baby. Whilst this mourning process continues, with its slow adjustment to the loss of the baby one wanted, the real baby – the handicapped one – is lying there in its place, and requiring normal care.

The way in which the parents adjust to this apparently disastrous situation is crucial for the future welfare not only of the handicapped child, but of the whole family. It is not surprising that many parents are ambivalent about the child; that is, they sometimes feel they love him as if he were normal, and at other times still feel distressed, anxious, and even rejecting. This is because they love and want the child, but do not want, and are distressed by, the handicaps. They may try to solve this problem by "shopping around" for a doctor or hospital which will offer a miraculous cure. Parents who suffer severe guilt may attempt to relieve their distress, and to right the wrongs done to the innocent child, by one of two ways: they may either punish themselves by dedicating their whole life to unremitting slavery in caring for the child, or they may project the guilt onto their doctors, social workers and teachers, and angrily accuse them of neglect or mistakes. Sometimes they do both.

The reason that satisfactory adjustment must be rapidly achieved is because otherwise the handicapped child will become further handicapped and the family's happiness and social life partly or totally destroyed.

Without skilled help most distressed parents will tend to make an adjustment which reduces their distress, but at the cost of distorting their relationships with the handicapped child and the rest of the family. Ideally these relationships should remain emotionally and socially normal, but extra skills are needed to help the child overcome, as far as is possible, his handicaps.

This means that the child needs to be loved and accepted as a *normal* child would be – accepted as he is, with his handicaps, whatever they may be. Acceptance in the normal way, so that mutually enjoyable relationships are established between the child and his family, will allow the child's personality to grow in the most favourable environment. In the long run, it is the ability to face the world with self-confidence, to be friendly, helpful and useful, so that one is socially acceptable, that matters, not being physically perfect or very intelligent. Whether a child is *normal* or handicapped at birth, he will most easily achieve happiness and a satisfying adult social role if he is brought up in a happy, contented, united family. Even learning, in the strict educational sense, is greatly facilitated if the child is happy and secure in its first relationships within the family.

Adjustment
The first shock of being told of the child's handicaps is greatly lessened if the telling is done skilfully, and with compassion, by a doctor who offers to help the family through the early problem period. Many families do not receive this help even today, but things are slowly improving. If parents find they need more help than they are receiving they should contact the Spastics Society, or the National Society for Mentally Handicapped Children, whose local branches may be able to arrange contact with the appropriate professional services.

As the initial distress lessens, the family must take stock of itself in relation to the task of doing the best for the new handicapped child. Perhaps the most important asset a family can have is a firmly united partnership between the parents. It is of the highest importance that *both* parents should accept their full share of the responsibility for the care of their child. Any tendency for one to blame the other, or to feel less involved, or on the other hand for one to accept the total responsibility, can be disastrous. Mothers are prone to accept the burden, and fathers to allow this to happen. Mothers nurture the child for nine months within their body, and are told of all the things they must do to keep their unborn child healthy, and all the things they must not do, to prevent damage. Not unnaturally therefore, they easily fall prey to feelings of guilt, or inadequacy as a wife and mother, and believe they have to suffer alone in caring for the child. Unfortunately, doctors often reinforce this tendency by revealing the news to the father seen alone, and leaving him to tell his wife as best he can, giving the impression that it is really *her* problem.

Ideally both parents should draw closer together, and support each other by resolving to share fully the problems and the joys. Fathers should realise what an enormous comfort it is to their wives if they can speak openly about their attitudes to the child and each other, and if their feelings can be shared. Parents should also try to realise from the beginning that *they* also have needs as well as the *child,* and they should not stop living as a couple. They still need each other's companionship, leisure time spent together and separately, friends and social activities, sexual enjoyment, and a loving relationship with their other children. Nothing less than a normal family life is satisfactory for the handicapped child, its brothers and sisters, and for the parents themselves. The idea of sacrificing everybody in order to care better for the child should be thrown away. The handicapped child who has over-burdened and over-caring parents suffers unnecessarily, and so does the rest of the family. At worst the family may eventually disintegrate under the strain. Fathers who lose their place in their family may resent the handicapped child who has replaced them, and may even leave the family to find solace elsewhere. Brothers and sisters may take their pleasures outside the home dominated by the imagined needs of a handicapped sibling.

No: the handicapped child has the same emotional and social needs as other children. He needs love but not smothering; care but not over-indulgence; and above all opportunities for achievement, self-control, and social growth towards an independent adult place in society.

Shame, embarrassment and social isolation
One problem facing parents, as soon as they have been told about their child's handicaps, is what to tell relatives, friends, and neighbours. The answer is undoubtedly – the truth. You expect your doctor to tell you the truth, and you should do the same. Doctors sometimes misguidedly cover

up the truth for fear of distressing parents, and parents often cover up in order to save themselves and their friends from embarrassment. Friends and neighbours are bound to enquire when you take the baby home from hospital, and failure to tell them at once of the child's disability is only to make it more difficult next time. Tell all enquirers, including your other children, as naturally as you can, that the doctors think that the baby has weak arms and legs, or is severely mentally and physically handicapped, or that he has fits, and that treatment has begun. You have nothing to be ashamed of, and few people will fail to be helpful and sympathetic. On the other hand, once you have told someone that 'baby's fine', you have begun to lie, and to build a wall between you and your friends. As time goes by it will be more and more difficult to meet people, who can see for themselves that something is wrong. They will wonder whether you know, and are too embarrassed to tell them, or whether you don't know, in which case they won't want to be the first to suggest it. Gradually you will become socially isolated, your embarrassment causing them and you to avoid each other.

Of course, some people's attempts to help may be a little misguided. Some may try to persuade you that the diagnosis must be wrong: "How can they tell at such an early age?"; or that "He'll grow out of it". You must let your friends be sympathetic, as they are trying to be, and then help them to see that wishful thinking is not going to mend anything.

If you tell people in this straight-forward way you will quickly have a circle of helpful friends, relatives, neighbours and shopkeepers whose interest, enquiries, and offers of help will be of the greatest support to you and your family. The alternative course, leading to gradually increasing social embarrassment; distress at having to face the outside world; and eventual social isolation and withdrawal of the family into itself, is harmful. If you maintain, and even extend or strengthen your social contacts, you will be secure enough to be able to withstand the occasional rebuff or hurtful remark from the few people who lack understanding, knowledge or sympathy. Let *them* be the odd ones out – not *you*. Don't hate them for hurting you – try to help them to understand. The natural and normal behaviour of parents of handicapped children in the community, is probably the greatest force we have for informing the public of their needs, and dispelling the prejudice and ignorance which still exists.

Accepting help

Parents of older children often complain that no-one wants to help. Many people will help however, if given the chance. Right from the start – encourage them. Don't be too proud to ask for help, or to accept it if it is offered. Don't keep putting off the time when you return to going out in the evening together. Ask a friend to baby-sit, and then go out and enjoy yourselves. If you believe no-one would want to help in this way; that no-one but you can manage to look after your baby or child; that no-one else could cope with a fit, or that you must always be with the baby in case something happens: in most cases you are already making unnecessary excuses. You are over-burdening yourself without benefit to the child, and jeopardising the future happiness of the whole family. No family can be happy with a worn-out, over-burdened, irritable mother (it is usually mothers who martyr themselves). Find some baby-sitters. Ask your health visitor, G.P., or social worker, if you can't find one. Perhaps the local parents' group organises arrangements for looking after one another's children. Explain to the baby-sitter what the child's needs are, what may happen, and how to cope. Even teenagers are capable of taking on this task (and often very willingly), given the chance. The community will never really understand the problems of the handicapped or be sympathetic and helpful, if they're not given the chance to help.

Social acceptance – the ultimate objective
When the parents have reached the stage when their distress is diminishing and they have resolved to do everything in their power to help the child, it is time to think carefully about what one is trying to do. The handicapped child is going to become an adult. As an adult his happiness will depend on his social acceptance. If he has friends, can live and work in the community, and move about enjoying leisure pursuits and participating in community activities – he will be happy. If on the other hand, he has no friends, and he is shunned by acquaintances and strangers alike because his behaviour is odd, infantile, aggressive or unpleasant – he will be unhappy. Nothing is more important for the parents than to realise at the beginning, and to remember all along, that the ultimate objective in rearing your child is to produce an adult who behaves like other adults, as far as this is possible with disabilities – and it is certainly far more possible than most people believe. Any form of bizarre behaviour, especially behaviour which is inappropriate to his age, will make real social acceptance difficult or impossible.

But, you may ask, what if the child is not intelligent enough to understand how he should behave? The answer is – do not believe it, because it is never true. Socially appropriate behaviour requires very little intelligence for its learning. It requires only consistent training which provides the child with clear-cut learning situations in which he is left in no doubt as to what is expected.

Establishing the first relationships
Social acceptance begins in the family group, where the child will establish his first, and most important, relationships. These experiences will colour his relationships with other people, and personality growth will be facilitated if the early social experiences are satisfactory. The handicapped child needs, from an emotional and social point of view, exactly the same as other children. He needs love and care, but not *more* love and care. He certainly does not need pitying, over-sentimental, clinging, smothering, tear-washed over-protective stroking and cuddling

16

situations for the rest of his life. At first, of course, he needs lots of physical contact, lots of gentle vocal stimulation, and total physical care. But even this is not likely to be satisfactory, unless the baby is loved in a relaxed, joyful, accepting way, because babies are very sensitive to the mood of the mother, transmitted through her voice and physical handling.

Very quickly, however, the baby begins to establish himself as a person in his own right. He is not just helpless and passive, and if he is handicapped it is very important to observe and notice the little signs that he is beginning to listen and look, and to expect familiar experiences to be repeated. He is beginning to learn about you and the world, already!

The Changing Relationship
It is very fashionable to talk of child development, and to emphasise its importance, but few people talk of *parent* development, which is equally important. It should be obvious that the *normal* parent-child relationship is constantly changing as time passes. What is appropriate parental behaviour for a two-week baby is not appropriate for an infant of six months, or even more obviously for a child of five years. Beware the tendency to say: "He's only a baby," or "It's time enough for that later," or "He can't understand". It may well be that these remarks stem from a wish to deny the handicaps, with a consequent tendency to "infantilise" the child, so that he is thought of as a baby (and treated as one) in order to explain his helplessness. Unfortunately such treatment promotes helplessness, so that the baby's development is retarded, even in areas where he could be making progress.

The more the child progresses in areas of development where he can, the more his remaining handicaps will be obvious by comparison, and it takes courage to be able to face up to the gradual unveiling of the true picture. On the other hand, to keep the child totally and uniformly helpless in order to hide his disabilities for a long time, is to deny the child his right to develop maximal independence. For optimal development of the child, you must be gradually changing your relationship with him, always gently encouraging every effort he makes to observe, to vocalise and to explore and manipulate the environment. Month by month and year by year he should therefore be learning to do things he couldn't previously do, and learning under your skilled and caring guidance. This, not keeping him dependent on you, is true parental love.

One day he is going to have to live without you, and even if he is grievously handicapped, he will be better prepared for the parting if he has at least reached that stage in social development when he needs and enjoys the company of others, and is not still emotionally attached to his parents.

The ultimate objective of maximal adult independence is achieved, therefore, by starting from a basis of security resulting from your warm, tender, stimulating care, and moving gradually and steadily, with your

17

encouragement of his efforts, towards self-confident achievement.

The Mother as Teacher

All infants need frequent, close and intimate contact with the mother in order to form the social bond which enables the mother, and later others, to influence the child's behaviour. The association between the feeding, warming and comforting tasks which the mother frequently and regularly performs in the early months of the child's life, with her actual presence, results in the infant starting to regard the mother as his primary source of pleasure. The mother's face, smile, voice, smell, and skin contact become highly rewarding and motivating. The infant therefore looks forward to this stimulation, seeks it, desires it, and becomes distressed if it is not frequently forthcoming. The fact that the baby's waking movements are often filled with the pleasure of contact with the mother makes him feel secure and wanted, so that a little later he can begin to investigate the rest of his environment for short periods, secure in the knowledge that she is close at hand to help, comfort or protect him if he gets into difficulties.

The importance of this process for the child's social development is obvious, but it is equally important for his *intellectual* development. Learning does not start at five years of age in school – it starts at birth. The most important teaching is done by the mother, usually spontaneously and unknowingly. The frequent and close imposition of the 'talking face' in front of the baby teaches him the vital skill of concentrating on one set of meaningful and associated stimuli, rather than vaguely scanning the world in general. He learns to filter out confusing and irrelevant sensations, and to pay attention to one problem at a time. He also learns to be alert, to think, to anticipate, and later to explore, manipulate and experiment. He does this initially by becoming socially responsive, as he derives much pleasure from paying attention to his mother's face, which in turn responds to him and thus rewards him for his effort.

This process is essential for laying the foundation for all learning. It is impossible to learn without paying attention to stimuli in a structured way. This means being able to concentrate on the relevant or linked stimuli, in order to discover the connection between them, without being distracted by extraneous and irrelevant events. The mother's face blots out the rest of the environment by its approach to a very close distance; it does this frequently in a way which nothing else does; it repeats the same pattern day after day, and yet it is moving and interesting; it consists of shapes, colour and the fascination of staring eyes; and it is accompanied by movements, sounds, smell and comforting skin contact. Imagine the contrast which exists for an unwanted baby, or one which the mother finds distressing or repulsive! He is left to lie alone for most of the time, not handled tenderly, not spoken to lovingly, and not frequently comforted. It is not surprising if such an unstimulated baby

18

becomes apathetic, incurious, miserable, and socially unresponsive. Little useful learning will then be possible, and no motivation will activate the baby to seek stimulation and experience.

Play

The importance of play for any child's development is well known, but even today few parents receive sufficient help in learning how to play with their children. Play can be defined as a pleasurable exploration of the environment. If a task is interesting and enjoyable it will be actively pursued without apparent effort. If, on the other hand it becomes boring, repetitive or too difficult, it will soon seem to be hard work, and require self-discipline, external pressure or reward to continue with it.

The essence of play for the child must be *pleasure* – mutual pleasure for parent and child. If the infant is smiling and excited by the adult he is playing and learning. At first the games most likely to give pleasure are simple physical contact games (cuddling, tickling, stroking, rubbing noses, kissing); visual games (approach and retreat of your face, movements of your mouth, tongue and head, hiding and reappearing); and vocal games (singing, gentle talking, lip and tongue noises, blowing and puffing air). These lead on to simple nursery games of a more structured type, such as 'clap hands' and 'round the garden'. We must not forget that fathers also need to play with babies. They play differently and more roughly even from the beginning. They talk in a deeper voice, look slightly different, and engage in anti-gravity play – see chapter 3, figs. 19. This provides the baby with excitement and variety of play, as well as getting him used to males and their different behaviour.

Noisy toys are useful – rattles, paper being crumpled, spoons banged on trays or cups – because it is vital that the baby becomes interested in sounds. Always talk when you are with your baby: never handle him silently. Don't try to get him to imitate single words – let him hear the sing-song rhythm of normal speech, and the flow of normal language. He will later on try to imitate this, and you will be excited when he 'scribble-talks' in his own 'language'. Even if his cerebral palsy affects the muscles of the throat and mouth, he will understand more by hearing sentences spoken spontaneously, than by listening to words repeated artificially.

When the baby makes a noise, imitate it – even a burp or chuckle. Then wait a little while and repeat the noise again. Later on the baby will listen for your response, and smile when he hears it. He is now playing with sounds! Still later he will make his noise in order to get you to copy, and then you are 'throwing' sounds back and forwards like a ball, with enjoyment. You can then vary the sound and he will try to follow you, and you are teaching him to enjoy learning to control his speech organs to make the sounds he wants. He is well on the way to acquiring speech.

The point about waiting for a response from the baby is an important one during any form of play or learning. It is all too easy to be too impatient, and to keep showing a child what you want him to do, without giving him a chance to try himself. By waiting, after you have shown the child what to do, you increase the desire on his part to act in an effort to try for himself. You make it clear to him that you want him to participate. If he tries to imitate your play or your voice, repeat the procedure and wait again, so that he knows it is his turn. The more handicapped the child, mentally or physically (or both), the more one needs to wait in order to encourage him to participate. Too much hurry or repetition too quickly may deter him from trying to make an effort. He may then fall into a pattern of being a passive recipient of your efforts, and merely a spectator.

Self-help skills
The same principles apply here as for play. Every effort should be made to encourage the child to attempt tasks for himself. This requires not only patience but *time*. He must not be left to struggle too long unaided, so that he is discouraged by failure, nor must everything be done hurriedly for him, so that he becomes a passive doll. He must be shown the task, and then helped to go through the movements with his own hands or body. After a number of trials like this, he may be moving with you, or at least offering minimal resistance. At this point you should gradually withdraw your effort, *particularly at the end of a sequence*, so that he completes the task for himself. For example, when feeding with a spoon, put your hand over his hand when holding the spoon. Then take it to the food, fill it, take it to his mouth and after a few trials withdraw your hand at the last point before the spoon goes into his mouth. The task is therefore easily understood, and *the tendency to complete the sequence is maximal*. In fact it would almost require a positive desire to resist completion of the task.

This process of active encouragement of self-help and participation must start at birth. Encourage the baby to look at the bottle or breast and to open his mouth when it is touched by the teat or nipple. Don't just force it in! It is so easy to believe the new-born baby is helpless and not able to understand, especially if you know he is handicapped. But failure to interest, stimulate, activate, and motivate for exploration is in fact *discouragement*. The baby is learning, whether you like it or not. If he is not being taught to help himself he is being taught to lie helplessly. It may give a mother a satisfaction to feel the child is totally dependent on her, and will always be so, but this is really a poor substitute for the joy of helping one's child to learn, to struggle, and to overcome his handicap.

Some guiding principles
During any teaching periods attention to the following principles may be helpful in making your efforts more effective:-

The baby, infant or child must be keen to co-operate, and therefore alert, happy, responsive to you, and interested in the task. Teach when he is most highly motivated, for example feeding is best taught at the beginning of a meal when he is hungry, not at the end when he is satisfied and likely to play about or resist.

The teaching period should be kept short, and ended at once if boredom or protest of any sort begins.

No battling should occur – if it does you will always lose. The session must be fun for both of you.

Demonstrate – wait – encourage – wait – demonstrate, and so on. Give him time to respond, and as soon as he makes any effort encourage him by smiling and talking.

Try to be *positive* – encourage every effort, rather than criticising for clumsiness, messiness, or failure to complete the whole task. Encouragement and praise for every little effort will help him to enjoy learning.

Gradually work backwards from the *end* of a sequence, that is, get him to do the last bit, after you have done the rest. Then get him to do the next-to-last bit, so that he is working into the area which he can already do, and so that he gets the feeling of achievement as if he had done the whole job himself.

If you meet rebellion, or negativism – ignore it, and terminate the session. Remember – the more important a thing is to you, the more likely he is to resist. Why? Because he doesn't like the pressure to conform to your wishes, and because it is so easy to upset you by resisting. *Don't let him enjoy upsetting you.* If he won't eat his meal – calmly take it away (and don't relent – he should get nothing till the next meal, so that it is clear that he upsets himself rather than you). Cruel? Not really – in the long run it is kinder to be firm.

You must have both patience and *time*. Unless the slow, handicapped child has plenty of your calm, unhurried time, he may be unable to respond quickly enough, and may therefore look as if he is not understanding anything. This is particularly true if he is physically handicapped, because his physical responses may be slow, difficult or even impossible. If his limbs are paralysed completely, try to develop another way of knowing whether he understands, such as head nodding for 'yes', and head-shaking for 'no'.

Keep on trying if progress is very slow, and look for very small signs of progress. If you give up teaching him, he then has no possibility of learning. If you decide he can't do it, he never will. Remember trying to learn to swim? For months one feels it is impossible, and one can't understand how people do it, then suddenly it comes, and one cannot understand what the problem was.

Helping now

It is natural that parents should worry about the child's future. They often worry constantly about this, and are preoccupied with questions such as: "Will he speak?; will he walk?; will he ever be able to work?;

21

what will happen to him when we die?". These questions should obviously be answered truthfully by the family's medical adviser, as far as it is possible to do so. But often they can only be answered in a very guarded fashion, as accurate prediction is impossible, especially when the child is very young.

It is however, most important that the parents should concentrate on helping the child *now*, rather than worrying about the future. Worry is *destructive* – it prevents the parents from making the best of present opportunities, and it is also transmitted to the handicapped child, who will become unhappy. What is needed is not even a blind acceptance of the somewhat vague prediction you have been given of final performance, but a realistic look at the child's present state of development and a determination to help him develop to the maximum of his capabilities. Nothing is so healing of parents' distress, as the certain knowledge that one is working steadily and expertly, day by day, to help the child overcome his handicaps. Progress, even very slow progress, keeps hope alive – realistic hope for another small step in his achievement. Read, listen, and learn from others about ways of helping your child. You are his principal teacher and therapist. The professionals help, but they cannot do your job. Learn from them so that your child gets expert help all the time, not just for a few hours a week. And don't forget that you did the most expert and important job of all at the beginning, when he was a baby – you taught him to love people, to concentrate, to be curious, to explore the environment, to learn.

Concentrate therefore on the present stage of development and what needs to be done to reach the next stage – not on whether he will ever be completely normal. Regrets, recriminations, worry, sentimental sympathy, or painful longing for miracles, are not helpful. Effort is needed: informed, skilled, patient, determined, but relaxed effort, and not an excessive preoccupation with the child to the exclusion of your happiness and that of the family.

The task facing parents is like that of a mountaineer determined to scale Everest. He wants to reach the summit but he knows well that many have failed, and that he may fail. But he also knows that it is dangerous not to concentrate on his present position, and how to overcome the immediate obstacles in front of him. He may not succeed in reaching the top, but only a meticulous and careful step-by-step approach will ensure that he gets as far as is humanly possible in the circumstances.

Discipline
This may sound like a severe and inappropriate subject for discussion in relation to handicapped children, but it is not. Handicapped children must develop socially appropriate behaviour like everybody else, and they must learn that inconsiderate behaviour causes social disapproval. Even severely mentally-handicapped people can learn to behave normally in

22

social situations, because the learning of simple social behaviour requires little intelligence. It does however, require consistent behaviour by the adults teaching the developing child, so that he is in no doubt as to what is expected of him. If the handicapped older child or adult still behaves in an infantile fashion it is not because he couldn't learn to behave like an adult, but because he was taught to remain childish. Sitting still rather than running restlessly about; being quiet rather than noisy; leaving things alone rather than touching objects, pulling them down or knocking them over; co-operating with others rather than attacking them; playing with other children rather than stealing their toys: all of these are largely *learned*, one way or the other.

Discipline, or self-control, is learned gradually and begins early. Try not to think "He can't understand," but instead say to yourself "He's got to learn like other children". Right from the start the infant will begin to form that all-important relationship with his parents which leads him to seek your approval, and to avoid disapproval. This is all that is required for the infant to learn which behaviour is acceptable, and which is non-acceptable. Disapproval shown by the frown or scowl, and the more severe voice, should be enough to produce inhibition of the forbidden behaviour, and a desire to be restored to a position of obvious friendship. Thus distraction into a more desirable activity is readily achieved, with encouragement facilitating the change.

This process is, of course, used by most parents, but it can easily appear to fail, usually because it is not being properly applied. It only works if the proportion of approval to disapproval is high, so that the child can form a satisfying relationship on the basis of many mutually enjoyed activities. He then knows he is loved, and in turn he loves you – you both wish to please each other as much as possible. He will therefore, at least most of the time, try to avoid doing what displeases you. If, however, he feels that he is always, or very frequently, displeasing you, so that every time you see him move or hear him call out you disapprove, the relationship will clearly be mutually painful and disturbing. He will feel unwanted and unloved. Constant criticism and disapproval will cause retaliation, or withdrawal, or both.

He may therefore become increasingly naughty and enjoy upsetting or annoying you in one case, or take avoiding action in a fearful, timid way in the other. In either case useful social learning will not be possible, and the situation may deteriorate eventually to the point where the child cannot be tolerated in the family at all.

A child who receives approval and encouragement for say, 95% of his actions, and disapproval for only 5%, has the opportunity to be able to discriminate right from wrong. If the disapproval is *consistently* and *firmly* given in relation to particular acts or behaviour, these acts will tend to be avoided. Consistency means that *both* parents must disapprove, and the disapproval must be firm and unchanging. It is obviously confusing at best, and totally ineffectual, or even cruel at worst, if mild disapproval is followed by smiling or other encouragement, or if one parent is treating the child's behaviour in a contradictory way.

It is not easy to realise that one may be encouraging behaviour which is naughty, unrestrained, inconsiderate, or socially inappropriate. It is also easy not to realise that behaviour which is appropriate to one developmental stage is being prolonged inappropriately into a later age by continuing encouragement, when the normal process would entail a gradual cessation of encouragement, followed by the slow development of actual disapproval. Children cannot develop normally unless their parents develop, by which I mean that the parents' behaviour must 'grow up' with the child. In fact the difficulty faced by the parents of a handicapped child can be summarised by saying that *the child appears not to be developing, and so the parents may not develop*, and if the parents don't develop, the handicapped child cannot move forward.

It is therefore very important indeed not to stand still in your mutual development with your handicapped child, so that you both remain locked firmly in the earliest infant–parent relationship, with no changes occurring. Behaviour such as scratching your face with his fingers, and pulling your hair, may be attractive in an infant. Its encouragement at first by parental smiling and gentle vocal response is appropriate for the development of the social bond between parent and child, and essential for the acquisition of movement skills and for the learning of body awareness. At a later stage, however, the child should learn to be gentle as he grows in strength, because he needs to become aware of other people's feelings, and he should be moving on to exploration of toys, objects, and his physical environment. This change is achieved by parental encouragement of these object-centred activities, and disapproval of disruptive behaviour.

However, it must be heavily emphasised that it is not *disapproval* which is the most effective means of training social behaviour. It is far more effective to continue to encourage, and to 'move on' in a gradually unfolding sequence, so that the child is not allowed to stand still in his development. The introduction of a toy to an infant, who has previously enjoyed only physical-contact games between himself and the adult, immediately changes the relationship into a triangular one, in which part of his attention switches to the toy. Encouragement of his interest in the toy, and his manipulation of it, causes him to move on in his development, so that he does not get stuck at the person-to-person relationship stage. Although he still needs adult encouragement he does not now demand one's full-time undivided attention, because he now finds the manipulation of the toy rewarding in itself. The parent is rewarded by observing a gradually developing independence, and an unfolding personality which can adapt to other people and other social situations.

Obstinacy and tantrums
The tendency to carry on letting the child have his own way is likely to

24

result in an excessively self-willed child. Eventually the parents may come to feel that the child should behave better, and then suddenly decide to change their demands. This abrupt, as opposed to a very gradual, change, presents the child with an unpleasant and frustrating new situation. He is suddenly expected to give up some behaviour which he has for a long time performed without correction. It is hardly surprising if he objects and gives a show of infantile anger, such as screaming or thrashing his legs about on the floor. If the tantrum meets with success, that is if the parent changes his mind and gives in for fear of upsetting the child, then tantrums may be used by the child to get his own way in continuing the former behaviour. Prevention requires a gradual expectation of changing behaviour as the child develops, and a calm firmness in insisting that he conforms with reasonable requests.

If tantrums are already established they may be difficult to control. It is best to ignore the tantrum and to withdraw from the child to another room, or if a group of people are present, to remove the child to another room for a few minutes until he has settled. On return to the group the child should not be comforted because of his tears of anger, but diverted to a constructive activity he enjoys, and then encouraged by smiling and talking to him when he is co-operating. If the child is relatively helpless physically, it is often enough to withdraw attention while he is screaming by looking away, and then to restore your interest as soon as he has quietened.

It must be pointed out, however, that if tantrums are well-established, the child will go through a period at first when he seems to get worse if a programme of control is started. This is because tantrums have worked previously in getting his way, and it is natural for him to increase his efforts using the hitherto successful method. He may therefore scream louder, and thrash about more fiercely and for longer, at the beginning of your efforts to control him. It is essential therefore to resolve that one is going through this period in order to achieve improvement later. If you give in again after a prolonged struggle, the situation will be worse, because the child now knows that, even in the difficult circumstances when the parents are trying to hold out, he can win if he goes on long enough.

It is also important that one chooses the time and place carefully to start such a programme. Don't start it whilst out shopping: it is very embarrassing to try ignoring a tantrum in a crowded shop or public place! Begin at home and avoid public situations until some response has occurred.

It must be emphasised that this rather fierce method, in which one seems to be exerting a harsh external control over a more helpless person, can be avoided by the gradual teaching of self-control from infancy, in the expectation that the child should be treated normally from the beginning. Ignoring tantrums (if they have become a regular feature of behaviour), coupled with placing the child away from social contact if the tantrums become fierce or prolonged, is still far preferable to smacking or physical punishment. The latter is not only more likely to destroy a satisfactory relationship with the child – it also teaches the child to be aggressive, as he will model himself on you. It may well lead to later fighting and spitefulness with brothers and sisters or other children. Nothing is more irrational than a parent threatening a child with: "If you hit him, I shall hit you"! This teaches the child that the bigger and stronger person wins, and not that aggressiveness and fighting are unacceptable forms of behaviour.

Obstinacy of the kind where 'passive resistance' is used should be dealt with differently. This is often due to the child having been under pressure to achieve, accompanied by much criticism. In other words, if the child is often criticised for being too stupid, or too slow, or for not trying, and the adult is impatient, irritable and frustrated by the child's fumbling efforts, the relationship will be unpleasant for both, and learning situations particularly painful. Refusal to try is a natural avoidance response, and at its worst is shown by muteness, a bowed head, averted or closed eyes, and clenched hands. Only by avoiding impatient, demanding pressure to achieve, and replacing it by gentle, patient encouragement of constructive activities can this situation be remedied. It often requires the intervention of a teacher, or some other less emotionally involved person so that the child can more easily start a new relationship freed from past painful experiences.

Food fads, toilet training, negativism
The more fiercely a parent holds to the belief that meat, fish, protein or whatever must be eaten each day to ensure health, brain growth, or intelligence, the more likely it is that the child will refuse to eat it. The pressure to which the child is subjected makes him rebel. The rebellion upsets the parent and battle commences – a battle which the parent cannot win. You cannot force a child to eat and retain food; if you try he may well vomit it all up immediately afterwards. If the pressure is dropped the battle ceases and the child may well feel he wants what everyone else is having. He has lost the motivation for refusal, namely to upset you, which is obviously very easy if you are over-concerned with the need to give him certain foods.

A similar situation arises when there is pressure to eat more. The child who has had enough will start to play with his food, and make a mess. If pressure is exerted to get him to eat more, or quicker, he may rebel in order to upset his parent. If on the other hand he is treated as an individual who knows what he needs, playing can be taken as a signal that he has had enough. The uneaten food should then be calmly removed, with no retreat from this position, even if he protests, so that he goes without until the next normal meal-time. If he doesn't protest, then he didn't need any more; if he does protest he will quickly learn to eat what he wants without playing about.

For similar reasons toilet training is another common battle-ground. It seems so important to parents that pressure is exerted on the child to oblige, and he soon realises that he is in control, and can easily upset the parent. A child who refuses to use his pot, or who sits on it for ten minutes and then dirties his nappy just after the latter has been put on, may well have achieved full bowel control – but is using it for his own purpose!

Both the above behavioural problems are forms of negativism, or refusal to co-operate with a too-demanding parent. If you are easily upset by his disobedience, he will enjoy disobeying. If you keep pressing him to do something, such as eating his protein, using the pot, or tidying his toys away, he will refuse to co-operate and prefer to be negativistic. He has a will of his own which he wishes to assert, and if you try to dominate him he will try to dominate you, and will succeed in these areas at least. In certain circumstances he has a right to say 'no' (many infants acquire this word before any other!) and he will if you keep pushing him to conform to an unreasonable demand.

Other behavioural problems

In a clinic children are occasionally seen who exhibit severe behaviour problems such as screaming at night, head-banging, hand-biting, rocking, or over-activity. The child who receives little attention, stimulation or social contact, will tend to occupy himself with body-manipulation, especially if he has partial or complete loss of vision or hearing, or in some cases is severely mentally handicapped. Many stereotyped, repetitive behaviours such as body-rocking, head-rolling, tongue-stroking, and complicated movements of the fingers appear sometimes to be substitutes for external stimulation and manipulation. They also seem to comfort the child, who may therefore use them, particularly after being distressed. They are certainly difficult to eliminate once they are firmly established, because the child becomes absorbed in his self-stimulation, and is at the same time relatively unresponsive to social contact from others. Trying to stop them by a direct disapproving approach alone is bound to fail, so it is necessary to substitute something more interesting and pleasurable. Once these mannerisms are established, only a long, patient, gentle approach to the child by one or two people, who try to join in the child's world rather than forcing activities onto him, is likely to succeed in establishing more social responsiveness and interest in the environment. From simple physical person-to-person contact games, progress can be made to physical games using apparatus (such as swings and roundabouts), and from there to simple object-centred play such as catching balls or rolling toy cars.

Physically handicapped children seem less liable to develop these manneristic behaviours or to become withdrawn, but if they do appear, or you feel your baby is unresponsive to you, it is wise to seek expert help

27

early, so that vision and hearing can be checked, and advice given regarding play and stimulation.

Other disturbing types of behaviour such as disruptive rushing about and touching forbidden household objects, are often a means of attracting attention. Mute children, in particular, are likely to develop some disturbing type of behaviour in order to attract the attention of adults, and if the child is physically helpless he may be forced to use screaming. It is common to believe that talking, picking-up, caressing, or taking the child into one's own bed, are obviously comforting to the child who is distressed, and relieve the distress. This is certainly true at the beginning, in early infancy, but the child quickly learns to use screaming as a signal when he wants the social contact. As time goes by, the parents get worn out with the noise, and having to keep responding, they try to break the habit, which causes the child to redouble his efforts. He therefore screams louder and longer, and the parent either gives in again, or smacks him in irritable bad-temper, and probably then feels guilty at causing distress, and so comforts him again.

A *normal* young child obviously needs frequent social contact with an adult, and even casual observation reveals that he signals to the adult every few minutes, by vocalisation, eye-contact (looking at the adult's face), and physical contact (touching the adult's arm, climbing onto the parent's knee), and that he gets a response from the adult. Unfortunately, the physically handicapped child, who has the same social needs, is less able to signal effectively by these normal methods. If he cannot move, and cannot turn his head, and sometimes not even his eyes, what is he to do? He does the only thing possible – he cries. If this works, he goes on using crying as his signal for attention. If he gets little response he may become withdrawn and apathetic.

The remedy is obvious, but certainly not easy. The parent needs to make a very special effort to keep the infant near her at first, and in a position where she or he can establish frequent vocal contact, eye-to-eye contact and physical contact. It sounds easy but it is not. *You* have to make all the effort, because *he* cannot keep making the demands on you like a *normal* child, and because there is less reward for your efforts. You also have to keep this up for many more months than you would with a *normal* baby, and this will need great persistence and patience.

Another very important point is that you need to be very observant in order to detect the tiny signals which your baby, unless he is very grievously handicapped, will soon start to make. If he does look at you, you must look back. Of course, you cannot sit watching him all the time, so listen carefully for little vocal sounds, and respond with your voice and interest to these, so that he quickly learns to 'call' you. If you don't respond to these quieter sounds, he will often learn to use louder and less desirable ones. Try to remember how frequently a *normal* infant or young child keeps on contacting its parent from minute to minute, and that the handicapped child has the same needs. It is tiring – yes; mothers frequently complain of the strain of responding to the demands of *normal* children, but nevertheless we have to recognise the importance of this response for the development of children.

The adult's response will therefore determine which signals the baby comes to use by habit, to obtain the frequent attention he needs for his social development. If he is using screaming, this indicates that his need for social stimulation is probably being insufficiently recognised when he is quiet, or when he makes the early signals of eye-contact and gentle vocalisation. He may not need *more* stimulation than you are giving in response to the screaming, but he may be having to 'shout' loudly before he is heard. In other words it is possible that he is being ignored unless he screams, and then he gets what he wants, so that what is needed is the social stimulation to be given *before* he screams. Ideally this is achieved by the parent's heightened sensitivity to the gentle signals which the baby gives. It may also be true that the *quality* of the social stimulation is inadequate. The response to screaming is often just a comforting, kissing, cuddling, caressing, or rocking. What is really needed, certainly after the first few weeks, is the introduction of play activities, and therefore 'peek-a-boo' type games should be introduced as soon as possible, and then the use of rattles, paper and other toys and materials, in order to encourage interest in the environment.

The child who is less physically handicapped, may, because of the same causes, develop head-banging, hand-biting, or disruptive over-activity and other disturbing types of behaviour. The more severe and disturbing the behaviour, the more certain it is that it will effectively 'switch on' the adults in the environment to pay attention to the child. The adult therefore tries to stop the child carrying out the disturbing activity, and in doing so provides him with the rewarding social contact he needs, and is almost certainly not getting at other times. Again one must *ignore* the disturbing behaviour as much as possible, and *most importantly* – provide him with more satisfying and interesting stimulation *at other times*. It is surprisingly difficult for adults to be interested in children when they are quiet and constructively occupied, rather than when they are noisy or disruptive. You must be *positive* in your relationship, like a teacher. You must go *to* the child to interest him, encourage him, and play with him, because you want him to learn, not chase him to stop him doing things you don't like, or comforting him only when he seems to be distressed. Ask yourself: "When do I talk to him? When do I touch him? When do we look at something together?" If the answer is: mainly *after* he screams, or throws ornaments on the floor, or bangs his head, then you are teaching him to do these very things in order to obtain your interest.

Over-attachment

The child who is dependent for a longer-than-normal time is in danger of over-attachment, especially if only one person cares for him most of the time. Not only may this make it difficult for him to adjust later to playgroup, nursery or school; it may leave him very vulnerable if you become ill and have to go into hospital, or if you die, or if he has to go into hospital for a period. It is important that both parents, and his brothers and sisters, should play a full part in the first year of life, and that other people should be in some contact with him from time to time. Being handled by other people should be as routine a part of his life as for any *normal* child of the same age, so that social contact is pleasurable and not frightening. After two years of age these contacts will become more important, and should result in a gradual widening of the child's acquaintances, so that nursery activities are enjoyed at age three to four without any trouble or separation-anxiety. If the child has been over-protected, and has therefore become over-attached to the mother or to both parents, the introduction to the nursery group will be painful and distressing to both, and this will further convince the parents that the child is too young to leave them, even for a few hours. He will therefore still stay at home, and the longer this occurs the more over-attached he (and the parents) will become. Again these processes of social development must be *gradual* so that the child feels secure with you alone at first, and then slowly generalises this feeling to more and more people and relationships. A clinging, over-protective parent does *not* produce a happy, secure child, but one who is anxious, dependent and frightened of the rest of the world. Remember, your child, like other children, cannot belong totally to you: he has a right to grow away from you and towards others, who must be allowed, and encouraged, to share his care and happiness.

Social behaviour rather than educational attainment
Parents naturally want a child who is physically and mentally handicapped, to be able to read, write, count and to make further progress in formal education. But *social* behaviour is much more important than intellectual achievement, whether for *normal* or handicapped people. For the mentally handicapped in particular, with limited abstract-learning ability, it is essential to concentrate on the fundamentals for social adaptation – the acquisition of basic self-help skills (feeding, walking, continence, dressing, speaking) and the development of a likeable personality, so that behaviour immediately evokes from others a normal friendly and helpful response. One of the most valuable, and relatively sophisticated, social skills, is the ability to put others at ease and to get them to help us or co-operate with us. To be able to approach people in a friendly, out-going, charming way in order to ask for help, or to offer it, is a great asset. Timidity, awkwardness, or fumbling, incoherent approaches, on the other hand, will usually meet with rejection, rebuff or humiliating amusement. This in turn is hurtful, and increases the handicapped person's social anxiety, clumsiness and misery.

This brings us to the importance of allowing, and encouraging, the handicapped person to help others. Full community recognition, as

30

valuable members, is accorded to those who are seen to be helping others. The helpers, the pillars of society, have the highest status, whilst those who are dependent and helpless – 'a burden on society' – have the lowest. It may seem strange to try to encourage a handicapped person to help others, but it can often be done. There are many mildly mentally handicapped adults who enjoy looking after severely handicapped infants and children, and who give them devoted care. In turn the multi-handicapped child gives the adult a loving relationship which they might otherwise never have. Both parties in such a relationship are able to help each other in a way which *we* may be unable fully to do for either.

Generally then, the handicapped person who might spend most of his life being helped by caring people at home, at school, or in a sheltered workshop or hostel, should be encouraged to give direct personal services to others. He should be involved in small responsibilities as soon as possible – for you at home, for his brothers and sisters, for neighbours and friends. There is no reason why the handicapped person should not enjoy helping old people for example, either at the personal and neighbourhood level or by taking part in organised community projects. We must not only aim at encouraging the handicapped to make their own decisions, exercise choice, feel the satisfaction of recognised achievement, and enjoy the same variety of opportunity as the rest of us: we must allow them sometimes to step into the helping, caring role that we have in the past carefully reserved for ourselves. Only in this way will they really feel part of the adult community.

Conclusion

It is a difficult task trying to write a helpful chapter for the many different parents of children of different ages with different disabilities. Some problems have been left out, whilst on the other hand parents may well feel daunted by the many difficulties which have been presented. It is better however, to have a quick look at the country ahead with all its hazards, before setting off on a journey, providing one is then determined to plan well in order to avoid the worst pitfalls. Being a parent is never an easy job, and none of us is perfect. Luckily children are very resilient, and most parents make a good job of their children's upbringing without instruction or much help. I hope, therefore, that after having skimmed rapidly through this chapter, parents will turn back to those parts most applicable to their situation, and then read those parts more carefully and frequently. If you still have difficulties which do not seem to be easily resolved, and particularly if you remain distressed, anxious or depressed, you should seek additional help. It may be that other parents will be able to help you, either directly from their own experience, or because they know better than anybody the best source of professional help in your locality. Whatever you do – don't try to press on in misery and hopelessness by yourself.

Chapter 3

MOVEMENT

If we are to be competent in appreciating and understanding the changing problems in the physical development of the cerebral palsied child, it is essential that we first know something of the physical development of the *normal* child, including the most important basic patterns of movement underlying future activities. It is also helpful to observe how *we* move thus making it easier to assess why the cerebral palsied child moves in a certain way and what is interfering with his movements.

Our muscles work in patterns, and the brain responds to our intention by making groups of muscles, not single muscles, work. The reason for this will be clear if you carry out the following experiment. Lie on your back and then sit up, you will find that as you lift your head with your shoulders and arms forward, your back will round and this will enable you to bend your hips and so to sit up. On the other hand, if you lie on your back pressing your head against the floor, this will result in your shoulders going back, the lower part of your spine will hollow, and your hips will tend to straighten. In effect, pressing your head back, automatically leads to other movements taking place at the same time in the rest of your body. You will fail to sit up because the grouping of the muscle patterns throughout the body are co-ordinated in the wrong way for this particular sequence of movements, and your body can neither prepare nor adjust itself to the desired movement.

This simple example is used to show that all our movements are connected. They combine to enable us to initiate, and then automatically to carry out, a whole series of movements.

The muscles of the cerebral palsied child also work in groups or patterns, but these patterns are abnormal and unco-ordinated because of brain damage. They cannot take place unless the child is able to use compensatory patterns, i.e. the movement is performed with abnormality and effort.

The cerebral palsied child, in common with other children, learns a movement by 'feeling' it and by trying it out. Whereas the *normal* child has a natural or in-built ability for adapting his movements to his own satisfaction, the cerebral palsied child is limited to a few and inadequate movements, movements that become stereotyped and on which he will base whatever skills he may acquire later. If, to begin with, a child uses

32

only faulty patterns of movement, he will continue to use them and perpetuate his original faults. This will prevent a more normal physical development, and the repetition of these faulty movements may lead in time to contractures and deformities.

The control of all body movements rests in the brain and is exercised through the eyes, ears, skin, muscles and joints. If, as is the case with the cerebral palsied child, part of the brain is damaged, development is disturbed and retarded at an early stage. The fact that damage can affect different parts of the brain means that, in some cases, the arms will be more affected than the legs, and in others vice versa. It may result in one child being able to hear and to see but to have difficulty in moving, or, in another child being able to move fairly normally but being unable to hear. Whatever the case, the child will start by using the abilities he has, however abnormal they may be, resulting in an 'uneven' development, as many of the stages of normal motor development will be left out.

For instance, if the child cannot lie on his tummy and support himself with his arms and lift his head, he may not learn how to hold his head up or to sit or to walk with a straight spine. If he can only turn to one side, he will not use the other side and thus his body will develop unevenly. If he is unable to bend his hips sufficiently and can sit only by rounding his back to avoid falling backwards, he will be unable later on to straighten his back when he is standing. If his legs are so stiff that he cannot kneel and crawl on the floor, he will progress by pulling himself along by his arms. His arms will then bend too much and in time he will have difficulty in reaching straight out to grasp objects, or to support himself on straight arms. If he can only stand up by stiffening his legs, he will then stand on his toes with the result that his legs will become even more stiff and he will be unable to bend them for walking.

BASIC DIFFERENCES BETWEEN NORMAL AND ABNORMAL SEQUENCES OF MOVEMENT

Sitting up from lying on our back
If *we* want to initiate any movement away from this position, e.g. sit up, roll over, the first movement is to bend our head forward at the same time as we bring our shoulders and arms forward, rounding the top of our spine. In this way we initiate or facilitate the movement or sequence of movements necessary for sitting up, see figs. 1 (a) and (b).

When the cerebral palsied child lies on his back we see that his head is often pressed back, sometimes his shoulders and his arms are also pressed back. He is quite unable to initiate the bending forward of his head and shoulders and the rounding of his spine, both essential if he is to move away from this position, see figs. 2 (a) (b) (c).

33

Moving away from lying on our stomach

If *we* want to initiate any movement away from this position, e.g. sit up, roll over and so on, the first movement is to lift up our head backwards at the same time as we bring our shoulders and arms forward extending the top of our spine, see figs. 3 (a) (b).

In this way we initiate or facilitate the movement or sequences of movements necessary for moving away from this position.

When the cerebral palsied child lies on his stomach, his head is sometimes pressed down and often his shoulders and arms as well. He cannot initiate any movement away from this position because he is quite unable to lift his head, straighten his spine, or to bring his arms forward, all essential if he is to move away from this position, see fig.4.

Rolling

If *we* want to initiate the movement of rolling, enabling us to move from our back to our stomach or vice versa, the first movement is to lift our head and shoulders while at the same time movement takes place between our shoulders and hips. We call this movement 'rotation', see fig. 5. There is in fact a degree of rotation in nearly all our movements, when we roll, get up from the floor, walk, or even when we reach forward to take an object off a table.

When the cerebral palsied child who is severely affected attempts to roll we see that he has no rotation. The absence of *rotation* is due to his inability to control the position of his head as previously described, and to his general spasticity, athetosis or floppiness, preventing co-ordinated sequences of movement between his shoulders and hips. Such movements as getting off the floor or walking are impossible.

When the child is not so severely affected (the spastic diplegic, hemiplegic, or the athetoid child with moderate tonic spasms) he will be able to initiate the movement, but with varying degrees of effort according to the degree of spasticity or athetosis; both the initiation of the movement and the movement itself will be performed in an abnormal manner.

When the child who is a spastic diplegic attempts to roll he can do so but only in an abnormal manner. He starts the movement from his head, trunk and arms in the normal sequence, but he does so with effort which tends to increase his spasticity. This not only causes him to over-emphasize the pulling forward of his head, shoulders and arms but also, at the same time, causes his legs to stiffen and turn in. The value of the rotation between shoulder and hips, in this case, is therefore lost, see fig. 6.

The athetoid child, as the spastic diplegic, has the ability to roll but also does so in an abnormal manner. He starts all movements from his

34

iegs, in this case increasing his tendency to extension of his head, spine, shoulders and arms, see fig. 7.

The hemiplegic child also has the ability to roll but will always initiate the movement from his good (unaffected) side. This reinforces the abnormal pattern of movement of the arm and leg (on the affected side) and means that he is continually orientating himself more and more to his sound side.

In summarizing it will be seen that, when attempting to analyse the child's difficulties, it would be a waste of time merely to look at, say, his head or his feet, if at the same time you ignore the rest of his body. You must ask yourself, for instance, what is causing him to hold his head in a certain way and what effect the position of the head in conjunction with the child's abnormal muscle tone has on his posture and movements generally.

When the child can do a movement but does so abnormally, we must again analyse how much of the movement is normal and where it deteriorates and the reasons why. The aim, whenever possible, is not only to get the child to move, but to continue to improve the quality of his movements.

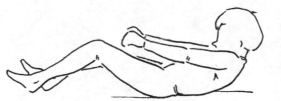

(a)

(b)

Figure 1
(a) A *normal* child sitting up from lying on the floor, raising his head forwards and at the same time bringing his arms and shoulders forward, hips and knees bend.
(b) Stage two, sitting up from lying on the floor.

35

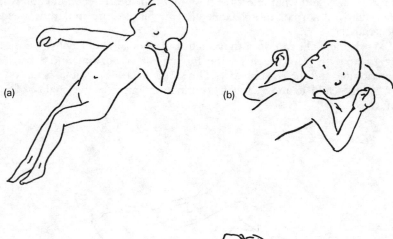

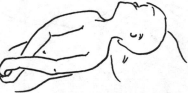

Figure 2

(a) and (b) Show the position often adopted by the *cerebral palsied* child when he lies on his back – head, shoulders and arms pressed back making it difficult or impossible for him to move away from this position.

(c) In this case, only the head and shoulders press back, the position of the arms straight and across the body will influence the position of the legs and hips making them stiff, the legs turning in. These postures will make it impossible for the child to raise his head or to bring his arms and shoulders forward and at the same time bend his hips to sit up, as illustrated in fig. 1(a) and (b).

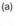
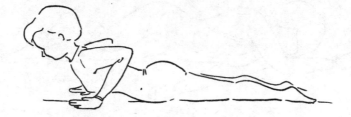

(a)

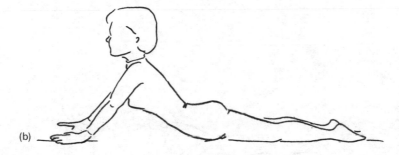

(b)

Figure 3
(a) A *normal* child rising from the floor lifts himself on his bent arms, at the same time lifting his head and straightening his back.
(b) Stage two, taking weight on straight arms at the same time lifting his head and straightening his back.

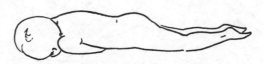

Figure 4. The *cerebral palsied* child lying on his tummy, his head and shoulders pressed down against the floor, arms tucked underneath his body. He is unable to lift his head, back and shoulders, or bring his arms forward to take weight on them.

37

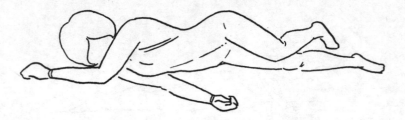

Figure 5. A *normal* child rolling, showing movement between shoulder girdle and hips i.e. 'rotation'.

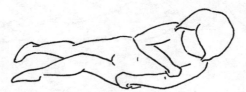

Figure 6. Spastic diplegic child rolling over, showing the effect on the hips and legs when he initiates the movement of rolling from the head, shoulders and trunk only.

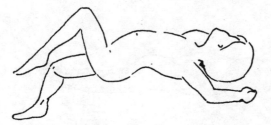

Figure 7. Athetoid child rolling over, showing the effect on the head, shoulders and arms when he initiates the movement of rolling from hips and legs only.

NORMAL MOVEMENTS POSSIBLE BUT ABNORMALLY PERFORMED BY THE CEREBRAL PALSIED CHILD

Pushing Himself Backwards on the Floor

THE NORMAL CHILD
At about eight months the baby, when he lies on his back, bends his knees, puts his feet flat on the floor, lifting his bottom to make a 'bridge', then pushing himself backwards, see fig 8 (a).

THE SPASTIC CHILD
'Bridging' is a movement seldom seen in the spastic child. He does, however, sometimes try to push himself backwards by pushing against an upright surface such as a wall, the side of a chair or the end of the bath. Unable to bend his feet up sufficiently to place them flat he pushes with his toes, reinforcing his tendency to have stiff legs and hips which, if permitted, will result in the child being unable to stand or walk other than on his toes.

THE ATHETOID CHILD
The athetoid child, whose legs are less affected than his arms, often finds that the only way in which he can move around the house is to make a 'bridge' and to push himself backwards. The movements of his legs and hips are similar to those of the *normal* child but, as he arches his back, he also pushes his head and shoulders back at the same time. This abnormal pattern will increase his general tendency to extension and retraction of his head, shoulders and arms. If persisted in this abnormal pattern will prevent him later from lifting his head in order to sit up, also from reaching forward with his arms and hands and taking weight on extended arms, and eventually from sitting or balancing in any position, see figs 8 (b) (c).

An *alternative* to abnormal 'bridging' and pushing backwards on the floor is rolling.

It is best to encourage both the spastic child and the athetoid child to get as good a pattern of rolling as possible. Your therapist will assess, with you, the reasons why your child has difficulties in rolling and will tell you how to facilitate this movement.

Creeping on his Tummy
THE NORMAL CHILD
A normal child at about eight months moves on his tummy by pushing himself backwards with his arms and by pivoting. Later he pulls himself forwards on his tummy by using his arms in a 'swimming' movement and pushing with alternate legs, see fig. 9 noting that, at this stage, his head and spine are extended and each arm and leg is used alternately – his forward progress is helped by pushing with his toes.

THE SPASTIC DIPLEGIC CHILD

Look at fig. 10 and compare the posture of the *normal* child when creeping with that of the spastic diplegic child, who can only move along the floor by 'pulling' with his arms. The pulling of the arms down and across the chest will gradually lead to stiff extension and crossing of the legs and feet, making it impossible for him later to stand with his legs apart and with his feet flat on the ground.

THE ATHETOID CHILD

The athetoid child is generally incapable of creeping or crawling as he cannot lift or hold up his head and cannot take sufficient weight on his arms when lying on his tummy. Therefore he can only move by rolling abnormally or by pushing himself along on his back.

It will therefore be seen that the jerky, uncontrolled and disorganised movements of the athetoid child are just as great a handicap to him as are the limited movements of the spastic child when trying to creep.

An alternative and effective way to encourage the spastic diplegic or athetoid child to move around the floor is in the 'sitting' position, as illustrated in figs. 11 (a) (b). Moving in this way means that the child is encouraged to take weight on extended arms, keeping his head and trunk extended, the continuous movement between the hips and the legs, while at the same time the arms remain still, is excellent for the child. He moves himself by pushing backwards with his heels on the floor while at the same time he straightens his legs, his bottom passing backwards through his arms, see fig. 11 (a). He moves forwards by placing his feet flat on the floor while at the same time he bends his legs, his bottom passing forwards through his arms, see fig. 11 (b). He can move sideways and turn using the same combination of movements.

The difficulties that face the child trying to do such a movement vary and should be carefully analysed. The child should start by first sitting in the initial position, i.e. sitting with bent hips and legs with his feet flat on the floor and arms straight. He then learns to move his head independently of his body and limbs. Sitting against the wall is a good way to start learning to hold this position.

Another way for the athetoid child to move around, and which should be encouraged, is to let him lie on the roller board, see page 192. This will help him to bring his arms forward, learning to take weight on both hands as he pushes himself around, at the same time encouraging him to lift and control his head, extending his back, a pattern that he will need later when he sits, stands and walks. The young spastic child can also get around on a roller board, but it is important to see that he has something between his legs and that the effort of propelling himself around does not result in his legs becoming stiff and turning in.

As soon as both groups of children have sitting balance get them off the floor using the modified roller seat, the small scooped stool, the wheel on rollers, or the tricycle, see chapter 14.

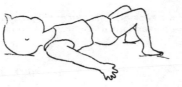

(a)

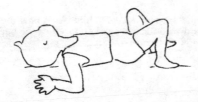

(b)

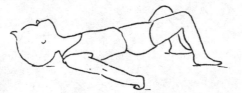

(c)

Figure 8
(a) A *normal* child lies on his back making a 'bridge', his head and shoulders remain on the floor.
(b) and (c) The *athetoid* child also attempts to make a 'bridge' but is unable to extend his hips completely and immediately pushes himself backwards – his head and shoulders are pushed against the floor the arms bent as in fig. (b) or stiffly extended as in fig. (c)

41

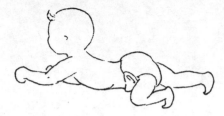

Figure 9. The *normal* child creeping on his tummy. Note how the head is held up and the back straight. He moves forward by using the opposite arm and leg.

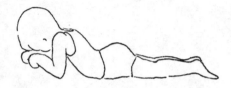

Figure 10. The creeping of the *spastic diplegic* child. Note how the pulling of the arms towards and into the body, bends the head and rounds the back, at the same time making the hips and legs stiff and straight.

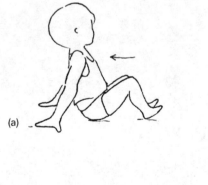

(a)

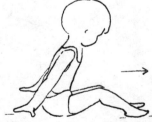

(b)

Figure 11
(a) The *spastic diplegic* and *athetoid* child takes weight on extended arms and pushes himself backwards with his heels at the same time straightening his legs.
(b) The child moves forward placing his feet flat on the floor at the same time bending his legs.

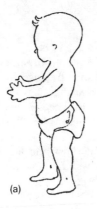

(a)

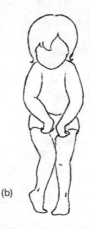

(b)

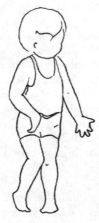

(c)

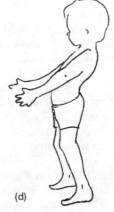

(d)

Figure 12
(a) *Normal* year-old child standing.
(b) The young *spastic diplegic* child standing. This posture is one of flexion. His head 'pokes' forward and up to compensate for the lack of extension in his trunk and hips. His arms are usually bent and press down and forward at the shoulders. His legs turn in and are held together, his standing base is very narrow making balance difficult and in many cases impossible. Some children do manage to get the foot of one leg flat on the floor as illustrated, but in doing so bend the hips even more and the whole of the pelvis is pulled back on that side.
(c) The young *hemiplegic* child standing. His posture is asymmetrical, all his weight is on his good leg. The affected arm bends and turns in at the shoulder which presses down and his trunk bends on that side. The leg is stiff and turns in at the hip, the pelvis is pulled up and back; his foot is stiff and the ankle does not bend, so that he takes weight only on the toes and ball of his foot. In some cases the head is also pulled towards the affected side.
(d) Typical position adopted by the *athetoid* child, his arms forward to overcome the extension of his hips and to prevent him falling backwards.

43

Standing and Taking a Step

THE NORMAL CHILD
The age at which a normal child starts to walk varies considerably but generally at about one year, by which time he has some balance in standing, if only briefly, and has reached the stage of starting to walk whilst being held by one hand. He balances at this time by keeping his hips and knees slightly bent, and by standing on a wide base, his feet flat on the floor with his heels down.

He is now capable, when held, of shifting his weight onto one leg, setting the other free to take a step, fig. 12 (a), shows the normal standing positions of a year-old-child.

THE SPASTIC CHILD
The variations in standing of the spastic child are many, figs. 12 (b) (c) show two of the more typical positions. It is obvious that standing on such a narrow base with the weight on the inner side of the foot, means that balance and the shifting of the weight sideways or forwards is impossible.

If you hold the child under his arms and 'walk him', all he can do is to fall forwards from one leg to the other, his weight falling more and more on to his toes and his legs becoming stiffer and later crossing.

One might possibly be encouraged by the thought that in this way the child is beginning to walk. Unfortunately this is not so, as the abnormal pattern of movement involved in this so-called 'walking' will simply increase the difficulties of the child in his efforts to stand, or later to walk. Other spastic children stand so stiffly on both legs, that even when you lean them forward they cannot bend at their hips to take a step forward.

THE ATHETOID CHILD
The athetoid child has difficulty in maintaining his weight against gravity, and when standing either collapses or falls backwards. For this reason he has no standing balance, and cannot shift his body weight sideways or forwards. If he is able to stand and if one of his legs is lifted, the other leg will bend and he will collapse, fig. 12 (d) shows a typical position adopted by the athetoid child to enable him to keep his shoulders and arms forward, hips and legs straight.

What is known as 'reflex walking' is generally present when a *normal* baby is born. Possibly a more descriptive term would be 'high-stepping', for when the sole of one foot of a new-born baby touches something solid, the other leg bends and then extends, giving the appearance of walking; this pattern of movement is also seen when a baby lies on his back and kicks. At about four weeks this type of reflex is no longer evident. If you 'walk' a young athetoid child by holding him under the arms, the movement he is making is identical to the 'reflex' found in the

44

new-born child, and if it persists will seriously impair the child's prospects of walking, because even the *normal* child learns first to stand safely on both feet before he starts to walk.

No alternatives are given for the abnormal patterns of standing and walking described, for although cerebral palsied children have common basic problems it is the individual variations of patterns that are of importance, your therapist, during the treatment programme, will advise you as to how to deal with these difficulties.

ABNORMAL MOVEMENTS WHICH ALL PARENTS ARE URGED TO DISCOURAGE

These are movements which, if continually repeated, will affect the ability of the child to learn more advanced movements and skills at a later stage, and may lead to contractures or deformities. One example only is given, i.e. 'bunny-hopping', as the subject is one that will be dealt with fully by your therapist during treatment. Parents will always be advised by the therapist which movements, if any – according to the child's particular difficulties – they should discourage him from doing.

'Bunny-hopping'. A method sometimes used by *normal* children for moving around, it is a movement often used by cerebral palsied children and one that should certainly be discouraged for the spastic child. The cerebral palsied child is obviously limited in his choice of movements and the very fact that he can move is good, but the way in which he does move must be watched carefully. 'Bunny-hopping' is an abnormal movement and continually moving in such a way will, in the spastic child, increase the tendency of the hips to turn in and of the hips, knees and ankles to bend, eventually making standing and walking very difficult.

Care should be taken to reduce the length of time in which the child moves in this way, and every effort should be made to encourage an alternative method of getting about, such as a child's motorcar, or perhaps one of the ideas suggested in chapter 14.

If the athetoid child cannot stand or walk, 'bunny-hopping' is permissible for a limited time, as these children do not run the same risk of developing flexor contractures in their legs. It is also a practicable alternative to pushing themselves along the floor on their backs. When the child has athetosis and spasticity 'bunny-hopping' must be discouraged.

METHODS OF HANDLING NOT RECOMMENDED AND THE REASONS WHY

It should be recognised that there is as positive a therapy in the avoidance of some movements as there is in the performance of others, provided that the reasons for avoiding them are clearly understood.

The following three examples illustrate how, by *our handling* of the child, we can inadvertently aggravate his abnormal movements, making the spastic child stiffer and resulting in the athetoid child having more involuntary movements.

Pulling up to Sitting from Lying on the Back
THE NORMAL CHILD
The child in fig. 13 has reached the stage of being ready, with help, to assist in pulling himself up to a sitting position. You will see that he is symmetrical, his head is in mid-line to his trunk and he has good head control. He reaches out to grasp one's hands and at the same time pulls himself up, lifting his head and shoulders off the pillow, bending at the hips, knees and ankles, a co-ordinated pattern of movement facilitating sitting up and the attainment of a good sitting position.

THE SPASTIC DIPLEGIC CHILD
The child in fig. 14, is a spastic diplegic. As you will see from the illustration, although he is fairly symmetrical and has some head control, he is still not ready to help when one starts to pull him up into a sitting position. He is unable to reach sufficiently to grasp one's hands, but he could manage to do so if he were allowed to keep his elbows bent; note that, as he is pulled up, his head and arms are forward onto his chest, he extends his hips and legs, turning his legs in and sometimes crossing them. If the child were to be continually pulled up to sitting in this way, his spine would become more rounded, his arms more bent, and he would be unable to bend his hips and knees in order to sit up.

THE ATHETOID CHILD
Fig. 15, shows an athetoid child. The child is not symmetrical, has no head control, and no ability to grasp. If one were to try to pull him up to sitting, his head, shoulders and arms would pull backwards, the spine would extend and, at the same time, the hips and knees would bend.

Here again, persistence will lead to reinforcement of the abnormal patterns of movement. The child may learn to sit, but only at the expense of excessive bending at the hips to compensate for the extension of the spine, head and arms. The child would not gain head control nor would he learn to grasp, hold-on in order to pull himself up to sitting, or support himself when sitting.

Bouncing on the Floor
THE NORMAL CHILD
Study fig. 16, and you will see that the child's head is in mid-line, that his body is straight and that his arms and legs are in a normal position – thus he is symmetrical. Note that as he is lifted into the air his legs are drawn up, they then straighten a little as he is lowered. As his feet touch the ground he momentarily takes some weight, although he soon sags at the hips and knees. Eventually, as he grows older, his legs will straighten in the air and his feet will be in a position to take his weight.

THE SPASTIC CHILD

Now compare fig. 17, which illustrates the abnormal position and pattern of movement of a severely affected spastic child.

Note that he is not symmetrical. The head is not in mid-line and his body is not straight. Note also, that as he is lifted into the air, as the head and trunk are not symmetrical, the pelvis becomes pulled up and back on the one side, and the hips and legs extend and turn in – in some cases the legs cross, his feet extend downwards, his shoulders pull forward and down and his arms bend and pull into his sides. On reaching the ground with his toes he is not able to put down his heels and takes no weight but pushes himself backwards. Compare this with the way in which a *normal* child takes his weight when we 'bounce' him. 'Bouncing' a spastic child on his toes will aggravate the abnormal postures and movements which we have just described, at the same time making his legs stiff. This will seriously retard the child's progress towards standing because, standing on his toes with a narrow base he cannot learn later to balance, or to separate his legs in order to transfer his weight from one leg to another to take a step.

THE ATHETOID CHILD

When lifted into the air to bounce him – see fig. 18, the athetoid child may straighten his legs but does not usually turn them in nor cross them. When his feet touch the ground, he cannot support his weight and he collapses, or if he throws back his head and shoulders he may stiffen and even cross his legs; he then stands for a moment on his toes and either collapses or moves his legs alternately up and down. 'Bouncing' the athetoid child will generally make him more stiff and increase his involuntary movements.

While 'Baby Bouncers' can be used for some floppy children or those children who are backward in their motor development, due to disorganised patterns of movement rather than to any specific abnormality of tone; we do not recommend the use of 'Baby Bouncers' for the spastic and the athetoid child as this will have the same detrimental effect as bouncing the child on the floor.

Throwing in the Air

For a *normal* child, throwing him in the air and catching him may be fun, speaking of the cerebral palsied child, do *not* do it *unless he is well controlled* – however much the child may appear to enjoy it. The excitement and stimulation will only make a spastic child very stiff, and an athetoid even more disorganised in his movements. We fully recognise the importance to the child of this type of 'father-play' but the child will enjoy himself just as much if you *swing him slowly in the air*, controlling him as shown in figs. 19 (a) (b) (c).

47

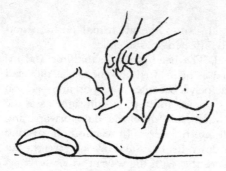

Figure 13. Assisting the *normal* child to sit up from lying on his back.

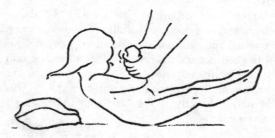

Figure 14. Assisting the *spastic diplegic* child to sit up from lying on his back.

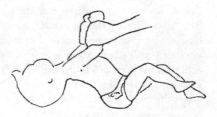

Figure 15. Assisting the *athetoid* child to sit up from lying on his back.

48

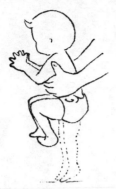

Figure 16. Bouncing the *normal* child on the floor.

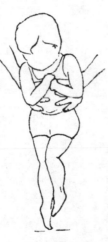

Figure 17. Bouncing the severely *spastic* child on the floor.

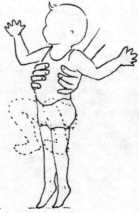

Figure 18. Bouncing the *athetoid* child on the floor.

49

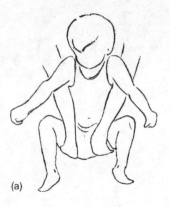

(a)

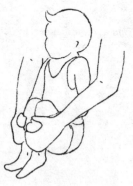

(b)

(c)

Figure 19

(a) 'Swinging' a *spastic* child in the air. His legs are bent and turned out by the grip illustrated, your forearms will stop his shoulders pushing down and at the same time keep them forward. Keep his hips bent and pulled towards you, his back forward and away from you.

(b) 'Swinging' an *athetoid* child in the air. The position is similar to that of the spastic but the control is different. Bring the child's arms forward, your forearms in front of his arms, hold his hands over the lower part of his knees. The legs should be bent and held together. Keep his hips bent and pulled towards you, his back forward and away from you.

(c) 'Swinging' a *floppy* child who has poor head control and a very inactive back. The legs are held at the ankles, the feet over your shoulders. By bumping him against your back, you will stimulate him to lift his head and extend his back and arms.

50

Chapter 4

BASIC PRINCIPLES OF HANDLING

As we study the development of the *normal* baby we see how the development of head control is the basis for all our movements and activities, whether they be automatic or spontaneous movements of balance, or voluntary movements; whenever we move we adjust the position of the head, holding it steady in mid-line to the body.

When observing the motor development of the cerebral palsied child you will see that not only is head control delayed and inadequate, but that the abnormal reaction patterns of the body stem from the head, neck and spine; it follows therefore that control of these abnormal patterns is most effective from these points known as 'key-points'.

I have illustrated in figs. 20 to 42 techniques of handling and some of the more typical abnormal reactions of the cerebral palsied child; there are, of course, individual variations of these reactions, handling at key points will make certain movements easier.

An important factor when handling the cerebral palsied child, especially in the early years, is the ability to use *our* hands both effectively and economically. You will see when studying the sketches that the emphasis is on symmetry and that in addition to the 'key-points' just described I also refer to other 'key-points' – the shoulder and shoulder girdle, the hips and the pelvis.

While learning to observe the child's abnormally co-ordinated patterns of posture and movement and their effect on the whole child, you must become sensitive to the varying changes of muscle tone under your hands, being able to feel the difference, for example, between an arm that feels stiff and resists movement, and one that feels light and therefore can be moved actively by the child.

A measure of the child's spasticity shows itself in resistance to movement. For example, when trying to bring his arms forward in an attempt to sit him up, the degree of resistance that you feel will enable you to judge the difficulties with which the child is faced, and whether or not the movement is completely beyond his power. In other words, we will know how much co-operation you can really ask of him and how much of a movement he can be expected to do. To appreciate the difference in the feeling between a movement of, say, an arm that gives resistance and one that does not, lift the arm of a *normal* person and move it slowly in different directions. You will realise how light the arm is and that there is no resistance. When you remove the support given by your hand you will feel that there is a momentary pause before the arm falls to the person's side.

Now carry out the same experiment on a cerebral palsied child. In the case of the spastic child, note the heavy feeling as you hold his arm, how it presses down and resists movement, particularly when lifted up, making it impossible for him to hold the position of his arm. The resistance offered by the athetoid child in a similar experiment, differs in that while there will be an initial resistance, the arm will suddenly 'give', but when you remove the support of your hand he also will be unable to hold the position of his arm.

The foregoing will serve to demonstrate the importance of 'feeling', in other words, the difference between the arm of a cerebral palsied child and that of a *normal* person. The same type of experiment can be carried out with other parts of the body.

In handling, as in treatment, our aim is to *take away* our support as soon as possible, remembering that where *you* are holding and moving the child, that *you* are doing the movement. You must encourage the child to move actively without help, he can *only do so* if you take away your hands at the right moment and then encourage him to move by himself.

It is important to remember when studying the sketches that whilst similar 'key-points' of control are shown for different children – spastic, athetoid, floppy – that the actual techniques of handling vary. Whereas the spastic child is stiff and needs to be inhibited while he moves, the athetoid child moving 'too much' needs pressure and stability and in some cases inhibition, enabling him to organise, grade and improve the quality of his movements. The floppy child needs pressure and stability in addition to other handling techniques to help increase muscle tone as the basis for active movements.

Points such as the importance of speed in handling and the gradual 'taking over' of a movement by the child are dealt with in the chapters dealing with specific activities, for example dressing.

I hope that it is now clear that by our handling we can prepare the child for function. To do this successfully you will need to learn, with the help of your therapist, to observe and to understand the reasons for your child's difficulties in moving and how these vary, to be aware how his abnormal patterns of posture and movement affect the whole body, and how by handling at 'key-points' you can influence or change these reactions. During treatment sessions your therapist will demonstrate and teach you the techniques that can be used to inhibit or increase muscle tone in appropriate cases, and how to combine special techniques of inhibition with facilitation.

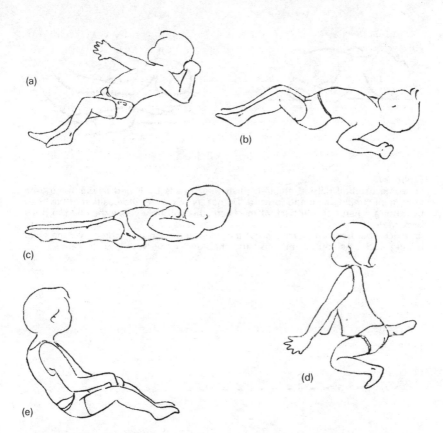

Figure 20.

Examples of abnormal postures, due to the position of the head, which affect the whole body. These postures will result in abnormal patterns of movement, preventing the normal development of righting and balance reactions.

Note: These postures will be more permanent in the *spastic* child, intermittent in the *athetoid* child, and seen on the affected side only in the *hemiplegic* child.

(a) The child turns his head, which may also be bent to the side, and in the very severe child pulled back. The arm and leg towards which the face is turned is straight, the hand open; the arm and leg away from which the head is turned is bent and the hand is fisted. This pattern is seen most clearly when the child lies on his back or stands and is often present, but modified, when lying on his tummy or in sitting.

(b) The head and shoulders are pulled back and the back arches. The *athetoid* child's legs may remain bent – the *spastic* child's legs will be straight and stiff. If the child is as severely affected as shown in our sketch, he may even show the same pattern when he lies on his tummy.

(c) The head is pulled forward, the arms are bent and are pulled over the chest, the hips and legs stiffen. If the child shows this pattern whilst lying on his back, it will be even more accentuated when he lies on his tummy.

(d) Lifting the head up and back, as illustrated, results in the arms stiffly extending and the hips, legs and ankles bending. Sometimes, as shown in the sketch, the child will sit between his legs.

(e) Bending of the head has the opposite effect, i.e. the arms bend and the hips and knees extend. This pattern can also be seen when the child sits.

53

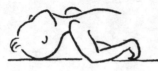

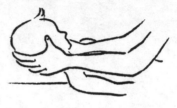

(a)

(b)

Figure 21
(a) Some cerebral palsied children push their heads back and at the same time bring their shoulders up and forward. Do not try to correct the position of the head by putting a hand on the back of the head, this will only cause the child to push back more.
(b) Place your hands on each side of the head and push upwards giving the child a 'long neck'. As you do this push the shoulders down with your forearms.

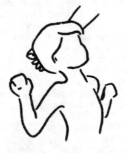

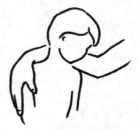

(a)

(b)

Figure 22
(a) If the child sits on your lap throwing his head, shoulders and arms back, do not try to push him forward as shown in this sketch.
(b) Illustrates a method of stopping the child pushing himself backwards. The forearm comes across the neck and the base of the skull, the hand and forearm control the shoulders, pushing them forwards and in.

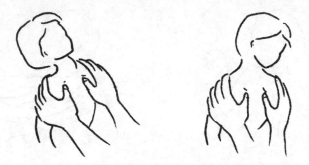

Figure 23
Some children cannot raise or hold their head up in mid-line because they are generally too *'floppy'*. By holding them firmly at the shoulder with your thumbs on their chest, you can give them some stability as you bring the shoulders forward, this will help them to raise their head up and hold it there.

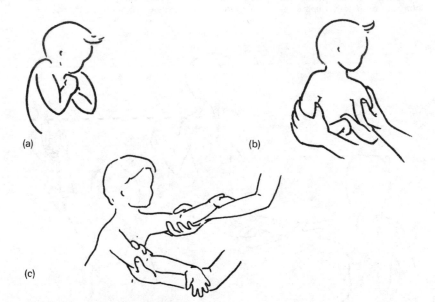

(a)

(b)

(c)

Figure 24.
These sketches show how by careful control you can correct the position of the child's arms and at the same time influence the position of the rest of his body. The child in each of the sketches is sitting.
Group 1
(a) A typical pattern of flexion seen in the *spastic* child. The arms are turned in at the shoulders; this is generally accompanied by straight hips.
(b) Hold the child over the outside of elbows and top of the arms.
(c) With one movement lift and turn his arms out as you bring him towards you. By handling him in this way, you can facilitate the lifting of his head, straightening of his spine and the bending of his hips.

55

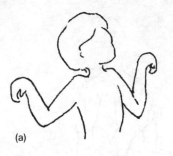
(a)

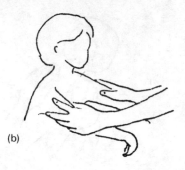
(b)

Figure 25
Group 2
(a) A typical pattern of extension seen in the *athetoid* child; the arms are turned out at the shoulders whether both are bent or one straight and one bent: this is generally accompanied by excessively bent hips.
(b) With one movement, the arms still turned in at the shoulders and slightly down, bring the child towards you and then gradually lift the arms up. By handling the child in this way you will facilitate the bending forward of his head, the rounding of his spine, and will modify the excessive bending at the hips.

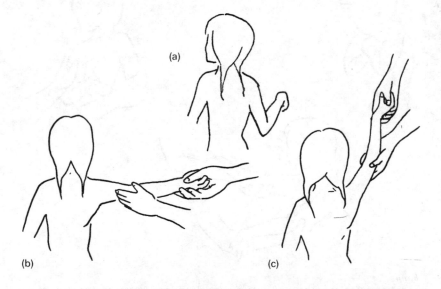

(a)

(b)

(c)

Figure 26
(a) Shows the arm of a *spastic* child turned in at the shoulder (which presses down), the head also pulled to this side, the elbow bent, forearm turned in so that the hand faces down, wrist and fingers are bent, the thumb lying across the palm of the hand.
(b) and (c) By lifting the arm, straightening and turning it out at the shoulder and elbow, it will be found easier to straighten the wrist and open the fingers and thumb.

56

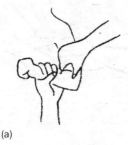

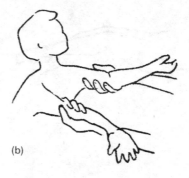

(a)   (b)

Figure 27
(a) Do not try to straighten the child's arm by holding above and below a joint.
Trying to stretch a limb in this way will only make it bend more.
(b) By holding your hand over the joint you can straighten and turn the limb in or
out in one movement.

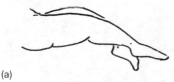

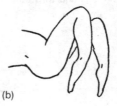

(a)   (b)

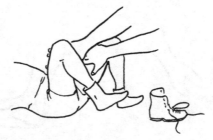

(c)

Figure 28
(a) and (b) Typical positions of the *severely spastic* child. If we try to bend the foot
while the legs are in this position, for example to put the child's shoes or socks on,
it will be found to be impossible.
(c) If the hips are bent and the legs parted it will be found that this position will
facilitate the bending of the foot.

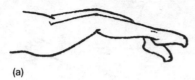

(a)

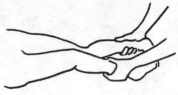

(b)

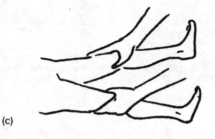

(c)

Figure 29.
If you want to part your child's legs and he lies as shown in fig. (a) do not try to pull them apart holding them at the ankle as shown in fig. (b) – this will only make him pull his legs together more tightly.
(c) Part the legs and turn them out, controlling the leg over the knee joint.

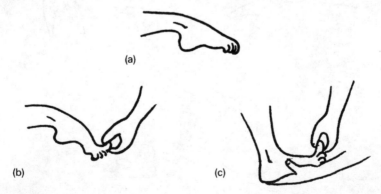

(a)

(b)

(c)

Figure 30
(a) The child's toes often claw (bend under) when the foot is in the position shown in the sketch.
(b) The wrong way to straighten the toes, as pulling in this way will only make the toes bend more.
(c) The correct way. First make sure that the leg is turned out, see Fig. 29(c), bend the foot up and then try to straighten the toes.

(a)

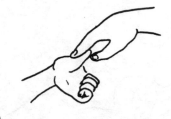

(b)

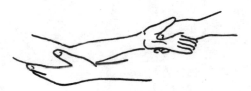

(c)

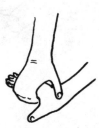

(d)

Figure 31
(a) Typical hand of a *spastic* child, hand clenched with bent wrist, thumb held across palm of hand.
(b) Incorrect way to straighten wrist and fingers – by pulling on the thumb in this way, the wrist and fingers bend more; there is also danger of damaging the thumb joint.
(c) By first straightening and turning out the arm it is then much easier to straighten the fingers and thumb.
(d) Correct grasp to hold the fingers and wrist straight.

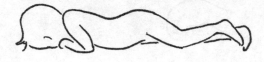

(a)

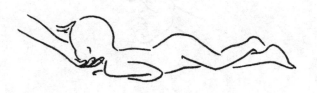

(b)

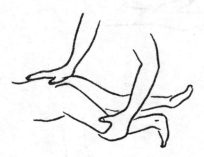

(c)

Figure 32
(a) A *severely affected spastic* child lies on his tummy, unable to lift his head or spine, or to bring his arms forward. His hips are semi-bent, with the pelvis tilted backwards on one side, his legs are stiff and semi-bent at the knees. Before he can be expected to move away from the floor he must learn to lie flat with his arms straight out in front of him and to lift his head.
When you are helping him to get flat on his tummy –
(b) Do not lift the head only, as this will only increase the pulling down of the shoulders, the bending of the arms and hips and will make his legs stiffen. Do not try to straighten the hips and legs by pressing your hand down on the child's buttocks, this will only cause the whole body to flex (bend) more.
(c) With one hand on the thigh, push the pelvis over until the child lies straight. Straighten the hip and turn and straighten the leg, controlling the movement over the knee joint as illustrated.

60

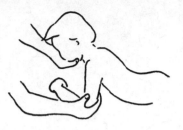

(a)

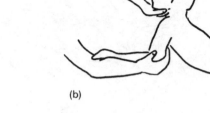

(b)

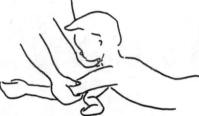

(c)

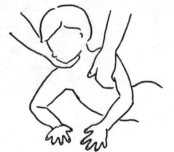

(d)

Figure 33.
The correct way to control the child so that you can put him flat on his tummy.
(a) At the same time as you lift, turn the head, start to bring the arm forward.
(b) Turn the shoulder out as you lift and straighten the arm – your point of control is over the elbow joint.
(c) Holding the head up, keep the arm straight and in the air, (as illustrated) until it no longer feels heavy and does not press down at the shoulder, and then place the arm on the floor. Follow the same procedure with the other arm. Do not let the head bend forward.
(d) If the arms are not too stiff, lifting the shoulder up and out with rotation of the trunk may be sufficient to facilitate the bringing forward of the arm.

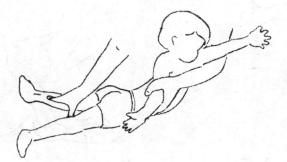

(a)

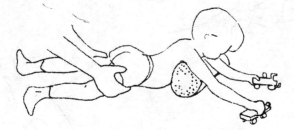

(b)

Figure 34
(a) When placing the child over a roller do not put him on the roller before you
have got him straight as illustrated. This will minimise his difficulties when he lies
over the roller. When the child tries to take weight on his hands or play in this
position, the tendency will be for his hips and legs to bend.
(b) This sketch illustrates how, by controlling the child by holding him at the hip
joints, you can keep his hips straight also his legs, and at the same time turn them
out.

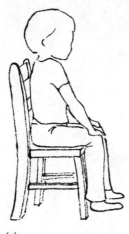

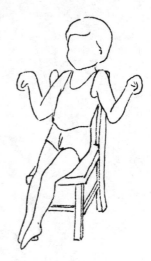

(a)   (b)

Figure 35
(a) The *normal* sitting position; the hips are bent, the back and head in alignment; the knees are bent, the feet flat on the floor.
(b) Illustrates the problems of the *athetoid* child with *spasticity* when he tries to sit. His fundamental difficulty is his inability to bend his hips, the reasons for this are:-
The pushing back of his head, shoulders and trunk.
The pressure of his buttocks on the chair.
The contact of his toes with the floor.

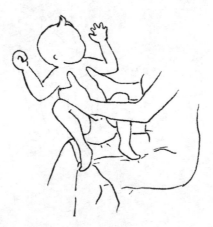

Figure 36. The young child with *spasticity*, sitting on his mother's knee, is still at the stage of having bent hips and knees (primitive patterns) but if held without adequate control the continual pushing back of the head, shoulders and trunk will in time cause the hips and legs to become stiff.

63

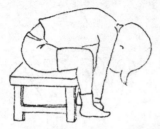

(a)

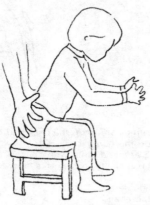

(b)

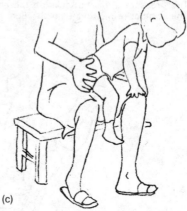

(c)

Figure 37
(a) *Floppy* child sitting, unable to raise his head and straighten his back.
(b) By placing both hands firmly (pushing down) over lumbar region (lower back) with thumbs at each side of spine gives the child a point of fixation and facilitates the raising of his head and straightening of his spine.
(c) This can also be done as the child sits on your lap.

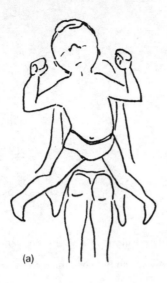

(a)

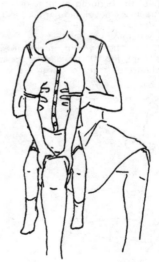

(b)

Figure 38
(a) Many cerebral palsied children have a tendency to straighten their hips and turn their legs in, even when sitting. Parents are advised in such cases to sit the child astride their laps. One should, however, realise that this may provide too broad a base on which the child can sit. The sketch shows the exaggerated position of a child trying to sit on too broad a base and points out the effect this has on the rest of his posture.
(b) The narrower base keeps the legs apart and the hips turned out, the arms and head are controlled from the shoulders, which are lifted and turned in with slight pressure inwards over the chest.

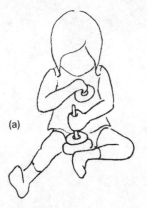

(a)

(b)

Figure 39
(a) and (b) Two of the many sitting positions of a young *normal* child. Note the wide base and erect spine.

The following are the reasons why we do not encourage cross-legged sitting for the *spastic* child.
1. Because of the bending of all joints there is a danger later of hip and knee flexor contractures developing, making it very difficult or impossible to stand the child later on.
2. It is an asymmetrical position.
3. There is too much weight on the outside of the feet which are turned in – a position of the foot that will develop later anyway in many cerebral palsied children when they start to stand and walk, we must try not to reinforce this tendency.

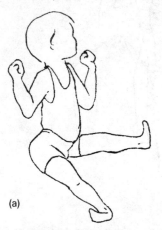

(a)

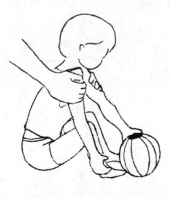

(b)

Figure 40
(a) Typical sitting position of the *athetoid* child, hips very bent with legs straight and wide apart, at the same time his head and shoulders are pulled back; this makes it impossible for him to use his arms for support or to reach forward to use his hands.
(b) The child sits with his legs bent and together, he is held at the shoulders which are turned in and brought forward, steady pressure is given. This will prepare him for the next stage, i.e. having his hands at his side and supporting himself. The same hold at the shoulders should be used.

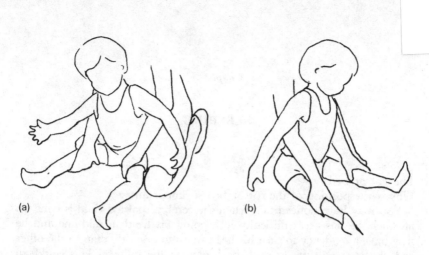

(a)   (b)

Figure 41
(a) When putting the *spastic* child in the position as shown in the sketch, first pull him towards you 'by the seat of his pants'. Never sit him on the floor and then try to bend him at the hips. The mother keeps the child's body forward which facilitates the bending of his hips and knees. She keeps his legs apart and turned out first by placing her hands high upon the inside of his thighs and then, as illustrated, holding him at the knees.
(b) The child learns to sit forward by himself and his mother helps to straighten his legs.

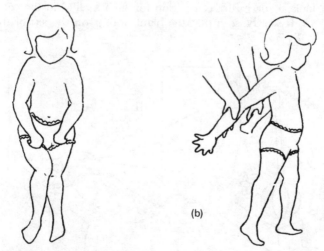

(a)   (b)

Figure 42
(a) Typical standing position of a *spastic* child. The abnormal pattern of her legs give her only a small standing base, her weight is taken on the toes or inner edge of the foot; this makes it impossible for her to transfer her weight sideways onto one leg to enable her to take a step forward.
(b) To help the child to walk. Straighten and turn out the arms held at the elbows, pushing the shoulders up and forward. This will help to straighten and part the legs and straighten the head, spine and hips.

Chapter 5

SLEEPING

The cot or bed
Why is the position of the cot or bed so important?

You may have noticed that when the cerebral palsied child is lying on his back, he has great difficulty in keeping his head in mid-line and he may have a tendency to turn his head more to one side than to the other and at the same time to push back against the pillows. This could, in time, result in deformity of the spine and the hips, the hip on the opposite side from which the head is turned tending to turn in. It is therefore important to take into account your child's particular problems before deciding the best place in the room for his cot or bed.

We shall illustrate the importance of this by assuming that the child *always* turns his head to the *right* with the effect on the trunk and limbs as described above.

First look at the incorrect position for such a child in the cot or bed, see fig. 43. It will be seen that the blank wall is on the left of the child,

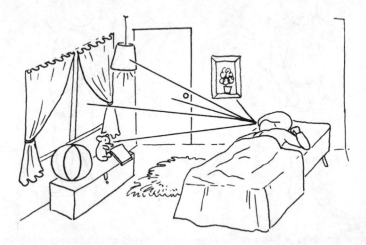

Figure 43. The *incorrect* position in a cot or bed for a child who predominantly turns his head to the *right*.
Note: All stimulation comes from the *right*, the window, electric light, position of toys and so on. Only the wall is on the left side; he has no incentive to turn in this direction.

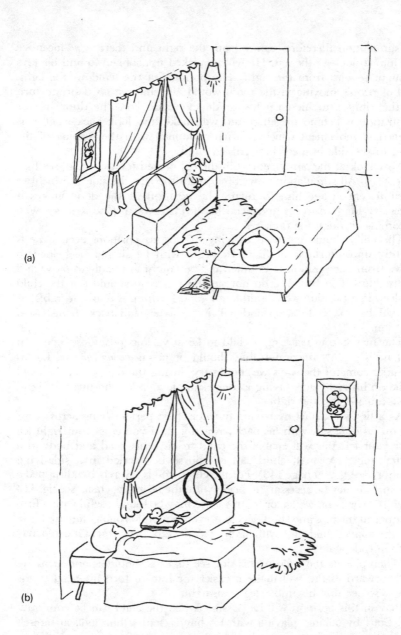

(a)

(b)

Figure 44
(a) and (b) are *alternative correct* positions in a cot or bed for a child who predominantly turns his head to the *right*.
Note: All stimulation now comes from the *left*, encouraging the child to turn this way; the only thing on his right is the wall.

all stimulation therefore, comes from the right and there is *no* incentive for him to look to the left. He will be picked up, spoken to and his toys brought to him from the right. The position of the window, the light, and of people moving in the room would all reinforce his desire to turn to the right and increase his tendency to do so. The door in our illustration is behind the child and will make him look back when it is opened, a movement which is often combined with the turning of the head to the side in a cerebral palsied child.

Now look at the *correct position* in the cot or bed for this child, see figs. 44 (a) (b). All stimulation now comes from the left, the side to which we want to encourage him to turn. The position of the door makes it necessary for him to lift and bend his head forward if he is to see who is coming through the door.

The child should get used to lying in various positions even if he is slightly uncomfortable at first. To begin with he should be helped to move from one position to another and be taught gradually to move and adjust himself in bed. We do not suggest that you should put the child to sleep in a position which, although good for him, is uncomfortable, as he will be unable to sleep and will immediately fall back to his usual position.

The first step in teaching a child to lie in various positions, even if at first he is slightly uncomfortable, should be taken *during the day*. Let us consider some of the ways we should try during the day to get the child to lie on his right side, taking as our example a child who turns his head predominantly to the right.

As a first step, start by having him for short periods lying across your lap on his *right* side with his back toward you. If you cross your right leg over your left this will enable the child to have his head and body at a better angle. A small child can of course be carried in a side-lying position (see fig. 99 page 143). For the child who is severely handicapped a soft surface may be necessary to begin with, the bean bag chair (see fig. 113 page 160) or foam wedge or foam square may be found useful with a firm sandbag at the hips and shoulders to prevent the child rolling onto his back. For the smaller child lying with his back against the back-rest of the sofa may be found adequate.

When placing the child on his side see that his shoulders and arms are well forward as this will make it easier for him to turn his head to the side, also see that his under leg is straight.

Play in this position will be possible when the child can lie comfortably. Start by talking, playing with his hands, letting him look at himself in a mirror, gradually introduce him to toys, preferably suspended to make it easier for him to handle them, see fig. 45, or use a magnetic or felt board, etc. and later encourage him to look at picture books.

Night time presents the parents of cerebral palsied children with some of their hardest trials. Many of these children are poor sleepers, which is understandable as they use very little energy during the day and spastic

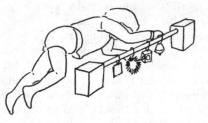

Figure 45. When the child can lie comfortably on his side, encourage him to play in that position. Suspending his toys will make it easier for him to handle them. Illustrated is a broom-handle which can be fixed to a couple of plastic or wooden bricks. Stops on the stick will regulate the distance to which the child can move his toys up or down.

children who are unable to move in bed become stiff and uncomfortable. We all move in bed, even while we are asleep, and adjust our positions repeatedly during the night. If you have ever slept on a soft feather mattress and tried to turn over, you can imagine some of the difficulties with which a spastic child is faced when trying to move in bed.

The spastic and the floppy child seldom moves during sleep and needs to be moved and turned frequently during the night, by placing a hard board under the length of the mattress a firm surface is provided, so making it easier for the child to roll over and adjust his position. Most athetoid children can move and are relaxed during sleep, some of these children move so frequently in bed that it is difficult to keep them covered. In these cases a warm sleeping bag with sleeves will be found useful or sew tapes to the four corners of the blankets and tie them under the bed.

Patience and constant training are essential if the cerebral palsied child is to be able to reach independence in bed, turning himself and uncovering himself, and getting in and out of bed on his own. Start training him as soon as he is capable of doing the necessary movements, and persevere. He needs to be taught what to do and have plenty of practice, or he will not acquire the simple skills which a *normal* child acquires almost automatically.

Help him to learn the sequences of movements he will need in future, while you play on the floor with him, for example, cover him with a blanket and in the form of a game and, despite the weight of the blanket, ask him to cover and uncover himself and to move about under the blanket and so on.

The following are some of the more common problems that may arise and suggestions as to how to cope with them.

Many children can sleep only when lying on their backs and in this position they have a tendency to press their heads back into the pillow,

71

while at the same time their shoulders and one or even both arms may also push back. This pushing back will have an effect on the hips and legs, making the hips stiff and causing the legs to straighten, press together and turn in, bringing the feet into an abnormal position.

If a child can lie only on his back he can, at least, be partially helped by wrapping a shawl or blanket firmly round his shoulders, keeping the shoulders and arms forwards and inside, in the case of an older child the forearms should be left free, this should help to counteract the pushing back of the head with its effect on the whole body. It must however be remembered that as this is a form of 'outside aid' as such it is opposed to our objective of getting the child to move independently. While this method may be useful as a temporary measure it should not be used permanently. The tightness of the shawl or blanket should be gradually lessened in the hope that it can finally be discarded.

The following are two examples of ways in which parents have managed to deal with the problems of children who are very extended when lying on their backs. For a baby *during the day* they have used a hammock attached to the cot, (see fig. 137 page 180) while he is sleeping, and *during the night* have placed sandbags under the sides and top and bottom of the mattress, forming a hollow similar to that of the shape of the hammock. A canvas camping cot was found useful for a child with severe athetosis and spasticity.

Some children have a tendency to turn in one of their legs while lying on their backs which brings the hips forward on that side. In such cases the child should be placed down on the side on which the leg turns in, figs. 46 (a) (b) illustrate abnormal positions seen in very asymmetrical children and a way by which this posture can be corrected.

Many young athetoid children lie on their backs with their legs in a 'frog-like' position. Placing a shawl or nappy around the child's shoulders and arms to bring them well forward, tends to bring the legs together and to reduce the excessive kicking of some of these children, see figs. 47 (a) (b)

There are other children who, when lying on their backs, bring their shoulders and arms forward and often tend to bend at the hips and knees when they are sleeping, becoming very stiff in this position, with the danger of the development in time of contractures of the hips and knees. When a child with so much flexor spasticity has learned to lie on his tummy during the day and to lift and turn his head when he is in that position, he should sleep in that way but without a pillow; it must be stressed that before allowing him to sleep on his tummy, he must have sufficient head control to *lift* his head whilst lying in this position.

If the child can *only turn his head to one side* it will be seen that the spine is curved and the whole of the trunk is turned and flexed on one side, this may give the impression that the child is lying on his tummy, whereas, in fact, he is not. Generally speaking sleeping on the tummy should be confined to the daytime as this makes supervision easier, or when the

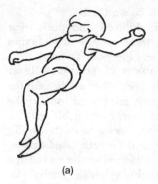
(a)

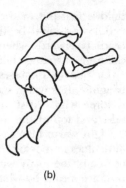
(b)

Figure 46
(a) Habitual position of some children when lying on their backs. The excessive turning out of the under leg, causes the pelvis to be pulled over, and the other hip and leg to turn in.
(b) By lying on the *opposite* side, the position of the pelvis, hips and legs are corrected.

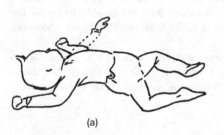
(a)

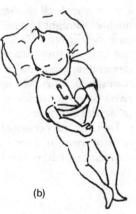
(b)

Figure 47
(a) *Athetoid* baby lying on his back – legs in a 'frog-like' position. The legs are turned so far out that the knees lie flat on the bed. The head and shoulders pull back. Two typical arm positions are illustrated.
(b) A shawl or nappy is used to control and bring forward the shoulders and arms of the baby. Top two corners of the shawl or nappy are brought over the shoulders and tied over the chest. Bottom two corners are brought forward under the arms and tied around the waist. Elbows and forearms are left free. The control given by the shawl or nappy may help to stop the excessive bending and parting of the legs and stop the kicking that many athetoid children do when lying on their backs.

73

child is first put to sleep at night and can still be watched.

Pillows should be firm and used only for children who push their heads backwards when lying on their backs, these are usually athetoid children or spastic children whose arms and legs are both affected.

Dr. Bavin discusses on page 27 the problem of persistent 'head-banging'. It is worth mentioning that 'Baby Bumper' pads are helpful for children who persist in 'head-banging'. The pads are placed around the sides and top of the cot and prevent the child from hurting himself.

Light warm blankets should be used as heavy ones add to the child's difficulties in moving. A 'tunnel' such as those used for orthopaedic cases, or one of the many wire supports that can be attached to the end of the bed, are means by which the weight of the bedclothes on the feet can be reduced.

Some spastic children dislike having their blankets tucked in, and can move their legs more easily if they sleep in the same type of sleeping bag that we have recommended for some athetoids.

Preferably the cerebral palsied child should be moved from a cot to a child's bed at the same age as would a *normal* child. Many *normal* children have a fear of rolling out of bed, especially when they first move from their cot to a bed, fears which are even greater for the cerebral palsied child, fears which can be lessened by the use of a very low bed, it also helps to stand a solid chair against the bed.

One problem from which cerebral palsied children often suffer, in common with all children for that matter, is that of demanding attention during the night by crying, asking for drinks of water or wanting to come into their parents' bed. Beware of starting to be taken in by any of these appeals, as they are the most common ways that children know of demanding attention and should not be encouraged. If you have already committed yourselves by becoming involved and are unable to break the habit or cannot understand why your child behaves in this way, do seek professional advice.

In cases of persistent sleeplessness and restlessness it is advisable to consult your doctor rather than worrying yourself about the many remedies you have tried and which have all proven to be unsuccessful.

Chapter 6

TOILET TRAINING

It is easy to become over-anxious when trying to 'toilet train' a cerebral palsied child. One of the mistakes most often made is to try to train too early, resulting in over-anxiety at apparent failure. The bladder of a new born baby is easily stimulated and is not under the child's control. In fact, some cerebral palsied children continue to suffer from this type of 'baby bladder' for an extended period, and training during this period will have little or no effect.

The *normal* child, until he is about one year old, does not associate his pot with its functions. At about the age of one year he begins to have some idea of the purpose of 'potting', and starts to indicate his needs by gesture. Gradually he begins to talk and learns to ask for his pot. When he starts to walk, he becomes so absorbed in what he is doing that he often makes his needs known too late. Nevertheless he is gradually improving, and eventually reaches the stage, at about two years of age when he is partially toilet trained, when he can manage to restrain himself until he has finished playing or whatever else he is doing, generally at this moment one sees him wriggling and jumping about. He will be about four years of age before he starts to take himself to the lavatory.

The process of toilet training is a gradual one, and can be easily upset by emotional stress, excitement, new surroundings, and during the first few days of school. Remember that the time taken to train *normal* children varies considerably, and is by no means easy.

Very often a mother will find that having, as she thought, succeeded in the toilet-training of her child, he reverts to earlier habits, these lapses are inevitable. She is then faced with the need to commence training again, a process in which a great deal of time and patience is essential. If it is so difficult to toilet train a *normal* child, how much more so is it in the case of the cerebral palsied child? Remember always to praise the child when he is clean or uses his pot, but do not make a lot of fuss when he is dirty or refuses, rather when he does succeed stress his achievements by telling him how grown up he has become. He knows full well when he has been wrong and getting cross with him will only cause him to be apprehensive and will not in any way help to solve the problem.

Ideally the best way of tackling the problem of toilet training, is to 'pot' your child at set intervals when he is at home, even though he may no longer be a baby, thus establishing a regular routine instead of one at odd intervals. Only frequent and regular potting will lead to success. Tell him why you are going to put him on his pot, and what you expect him to do; he must develop a wish to please you otherwise he will see no reason why he should not continue to soil his nappies. Always be within calling distance, giving him a sense of security, knowing that if he needs you that you are there to help him. Be sure that he understands that he is there for a specific purpose. There is always the danger of the cerebral palsied child being distracted if you give him toys, so as soon as he reaches the stage when he should be toilet trained do not give him anything that will prevent him from concentrating on what he is doing.

The greatest difficulty often experienced is the child's inability to sit and to relax, or to be in a position in which to be able to press down for emptying his bowels. For this reason the correct type of pot and its position is important, as also is the position of the child on the pot. As to the position of the pot, if this is placed on your knees the younger child will be more relaxed, and you can support him, which is essential if he has poor head control and no trunk balance, you can also hold his legs apart, see fig. 48.

A clear plastic is a good material for pots and avoids the necessity of lifting the child to see if he has finished; a small strip of foam rubber round the rim provides a firm base for sitting. A boy's pot with raised sides and something on which to hold in front is most satisfactory and will give the child added security, helping him to overcome his fear of falling. We recommend the potties that have a wide firm base and back support. See fig. 49.

A child will not be able to sit alone on his pot or on the lavatory seat until he has head and trunk balance and can sit with his hips and knees bent and apart, with his feet flat on the floor; he also needs the ability to bring his arms forward to hold onto a support. We have found that, as the child's balance improves, it is useful to place the pot in a cardboard or wooden box, see fig. 50, later the corner of the room or a triangle chair can be used, see fig. 51, always place a stool or chair in front so that he can hold on, or at least can have his arms forward, see fig. 52, which illustrates a pot placed inside a stool, a method which has been used successfully.

The potty chair, when needed, must be chosen to enable the child to sit in as relaxed a position as possible, but still with a stool or chair in front of him. Lately we have recommended the 'Baby Relax Toilette' and parents' reports have been favourable, see fig. 53. For the more severely handicapped child the wooden potty chair illustrated in fig. 54 gives stable support. This potty chair can be purchased from the Spastics Society.

The first stage towards independence in toilet training is reached when the child is able to let you know that he needs his pot, it is important that you understand the gesture or word that he uses to indicate his needs,

76

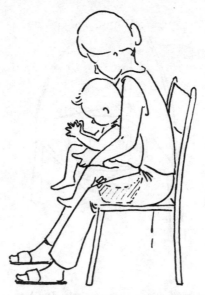

Figure 48. The pot is placed on the chair, the baby's back is well supported, the mother holds his legs apart, at the same time seeing that his hips are flexed, his shoulders and arms forward.

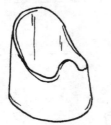 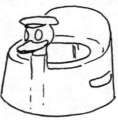

Figure 49. Two well-shaped potties with good back and front supports

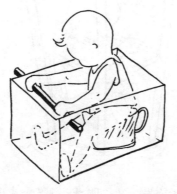

Figure 50. Pot fitting into a cardboard box. Bar to hold on to.

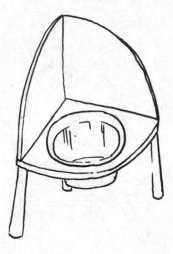

Figure 51. The pot is fixed into a triangle chair. The legs attached to the chair enable the child to sit with his feet flat on the floor. The triangle shape of the back of the chair keeps the shoulders and arms forward, this in turn facilitating the flexion at the hips.

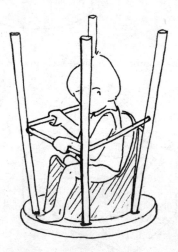

Figure 52. The pot is placed inside a large up-turned stool, giving the child a sense of security, the bars are well placed for the child to hold onto for support.

78

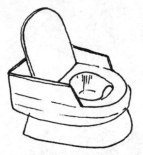

Figure 53. The 'Baby Relax Toilette' is an excellent toilet seat having good support at the back and side, with a solid base.

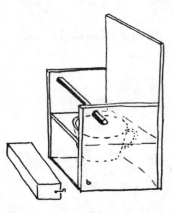

Figure 54. Example of a good 'potty chair' for the more severely handicapped child. Solid base, untippable. If the child's feet do not reach the floor, a narrow wooden box or block should be put under the feet.

also that you explain this to anyone else who may be looking after him. When he has reached the stage of collecting his pot himself, do be sure that it is easy for him to find that he can reach it easily. A boy, to begin with, can use his pot himself when kneeling, see fig. 55, complete independence will involve not only fetching his pot but also the ability to pull down his pants, to sit down and get up by himself, also to pull up his pants. In the first stages make sure that the child places his pot near a low table or chair so that he can hold on to the support as he pulls his pants up and down, see fig. 56.

The ordinary 'Kiddicraft' or 'Mothercare' type of lavatory seat can be used for small children followed, when necessary, by toilet seats made specially for handicapped children. Stools or boxes, one under each foot will help, not only to give security but also to allow the tummy muscles to relax.

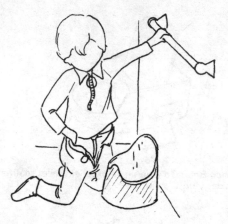

Figure 55. With the help of a bar to hold onto a boy can often manage on his own in this position.

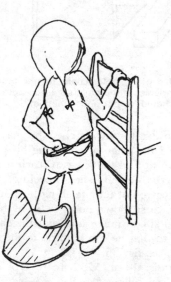

Figure 56. A solid chair provides good support while the child herself copes with pulling her pants up and down

Every means by which the child's independence can be reached when he starts to use the lavatory should be tried, for example bars at the side of the lavatory, and for a boy a box placed on a non-slip mat in front of the lavatory. An adjustment to the flush handle or chain enables its use without help. Finally do see that the toilet paper is placed at a height to which the child can reach.

General points to bear in mind in toilet training

If the skin of a cerebral palsied child is sensitive, to prevent chafing we recommend the use of nappy liners, such as 'Tufty Tails' or pads of soft cellular-cotton which are placed inside the nappy – two ways. Many parents find the washable waterproof tie-pants to be much more satisfactory than the popper type.

If, by the time your child is three or four years old, he is still not toilet trained, despite the fact that he knows he should ask for his pot, take him out of his nappies when he is at home, this will make him feel uncomfortable and more inclined to ask for his pot. Make sure of course, that at that time he is dressed in clothes which are easily washable. Trainer pants can also be used.

Normally, bowel control is achieved before bladder control, as it is obviously easier to anticipate a child's needs. If your child suffers from constipation, take care that this condition does not become chronic and if it does consult your doctor. Putting the child in a squatting position, or on his back with his knees against his tummy, for a short period of time, may prove to be of some help. Boys take longer to train than girls, both, however, will be dry and clean during the day, before your training brings success during the night. Do not start using a bottle for a boy unless his handicap is so severe that it is impossible for him to sit; use of a bottle is far too abnormal for everyday life.

The time taken to train even *normal* children varies very considerably and the whole process is by no means easy and remember that, the cerebral palsied child with his many additional problems will obviously require far more time, so do not be tempted to compare notes with your friends as the period of time in which success may be achieved is certainly not of major importance. If all your efforts to toilet train your child have met with complete failure, do not be despondent, there may be a definite underlying reason. For example, the arrival of a new baby may have made him feel he is not getting enough attention, or he may have come to realise that by you changing his nappy means having more of your time than if he uses a pot.

Parents are apt to think that only their child is slow and difficult to train, but this is far from the truth, toilet training is a very common problem with the majority of cerebral palsied children. If necessary do seek professional advice, as if the underlying cause of your difficulties is clearly understood, toilet training will certainly not be such an uphill struggle.

Chapter 7

BATHING

Bathing the cerebral palsied child is never simple. Although few difficulties may arise when the child is small, difficulties become more apparent as he grows older. The severely handicapped child will be unable to sit in the bath or use his hands for support, others may have the ability to sit but, having insufficient balance, will have to rely on their hands for support all the time.

In order to realise the importance of balance, think of yourself when having a bath. You will notice how much balance is required when lifting your legs to wash your feet, or the complicated movements necessary for washing your back. This will give you some idea of the difficulties your child will have in trying to keep his balance.

Baby's bath-time for you will undoubtedly be just another task in the routine of a day, for your baby however, it is a real opportunity for play and enjoyment. To combine this task with play and enjoyment for the cerebral palsied child means setting aside a fair amount of your time, it can however be time very well spent.

Suggestions that make bathing the baby easier
The best type of baby bath is one which has a slight slope to support the baby's back and is a good height for yourself, see fig. 57 and if extra support is needed a small pillow is now made with suction caps enabling it to be attached to the side of the bath. If the baby is to feel secure it is important to see that he is not lying on a slippery surface, a terry-towelling nappy is perfectly adequate, or if preferred a baby's 'Softie' bathmat with suckers underneath it to adhere to the bath can be recommended.

For the baby and the young cerebral palsied child the care with which you handle him *before* you put him into the bath is very important, the method described in chapter 11 dealing with picking up and carrying will provide a useful guide.

Some babies and young children have what is known as a Moro reaction. This reaction results in the child's head falling back, his arms shooting out and up, and his hands opening, this occurs if the child is suddenly tilted backwards, and makes sitting and balancing in any position impossible, and prevents the child, later on, holding on or supporting himself on his hands and therefore must be avoided.

The effects of the Moro reaction can, to some extent, be lessened by sitting the child in a good position with his head and arms forward *before* attempting to lift him into his bath, fig. 58. This position should be maintained while you are lowering him into the bath, rather than putting him in a half-lying position, as the difficulty of correcting this position when he is wet will obviously be greater. With a very young baby who has a strong Moro reaction washing him will be found simpler if carried out as illustrated in fig. 59.

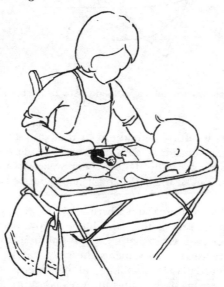

Figure 57. This bath and stand are the correct height for the mother and an excellent shape for the baby.

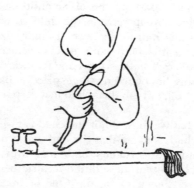

Figure 58. Correct way to hold a child who has a strong Moro reaction as you lift him to put him in the bath.

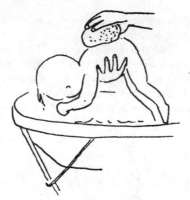

Figure 59. A simple way of holding a young baby to wash who is very extended, or has a Moro reaction.

The difficulties in lifting a child out of the bath are of course greater than when putting him in, as then he is wet and slippery; you will find it easier to control the baby if he is bent well forward from the hips before lifting him out of the bath, and if he is wrapped in a towel before you lift him out.

Play is a time for learning and where better to learn than in the bath? Suction toys for the side of the bath, hanging toys across the bath and floating toys, there is a variety of choice. Bathtime provides an excellent opportunity to repeat the movements the child has learned throughout the day, clapping, splashing, looking at his fingers, finding his toes, kicking as he lies on his back, on his tummy and so on. A cerebral palsied child often has poor skin sensation and faulty body image, and rubbing with a rough towel followed by play provides excellent stimulation.

Suggestions that make bathing the older child easier

Problems in handling may increase as the child grows older, for example when you start bathing him in the normal family-size bath, whereas the baby could be placed in a baby bath at a convenient height for you to manage, the normal-sized bath is deep and awkward in shape, therefore some parents at this 'in between' stage place a baby bath inside the normal bath, see fig. 60, or bath their child in a deep sink sitting him on the draining board.

The first thing that we must do, if the child is to feel secure, as we did with the younger child, is to see that the bath has a non-slip surface. This can be done by using an ordinary bath mat with suction caps. Some small children feel happier if, in addition to a rubber mat, they sit inside two rubber rings as shown in fig. 61. One of our mothers found her child, a scvere spastic, easier to bath if she sat, or placed her on her tummy, on a half-inflated ball placed in the bath.

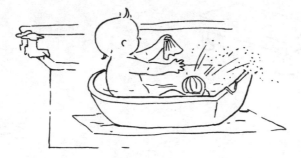

Figure 60. Baby bath placed inside a normal bath, water can be added as the child gains confidence.

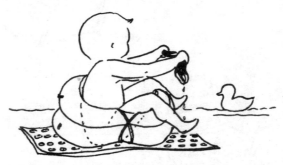

Figure 61. Two rubber rings tied together provide support for the child's back, and help him to remain in a sitting position.

Normally a bath is so shaped that the only way one can sit in it is with one's legs straight out. As long-sitting is the preferred position for the athetoid child, his problems are not so great as those of the spastic child, who finds it impossible to keep his hips bent if he has his legs out in front of him, his narrow base making his balance very precarious.

Types of seats that can be used in the bath
The seats illustrated in figs. 62 (a) to (d) are designed for the child who cannot bend his hips sufficiently to sit with his legs out in front of him, and also for those children who have no sitting balance. The 'Suzy Inflatable Chair' provides all-round support for the older more severely handicapped child. The seat is $13\frac{1}{2}''$ and the height of the back $21''$, it is anchored to the bath by strips of material that adhere to the surface of the bath. This chair can be purchased from the Spastics Society.

When you are deciding on the most suitable type of seat for your child, make sure that it is of the correct width and height. When we are advising our parents we always have a trial with the seat *outside* the bath, to satisfy ourselves that it is not only comfortable for the child, but also to make sure that it presents no problems in handling for the mother.

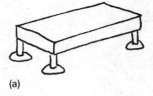

(a)

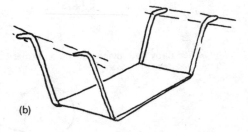

(b)

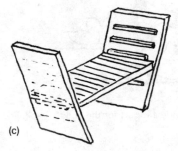

(c)

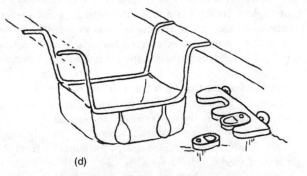

(d)

Figure 62. Various types of seats that can be bought or made for use in the bath.
(a) Simple stool with suction cups on the legs, seat covered with terry-towelling or rubber.
(b) Bath seat that can be bought at most large stores.
(c) Two pieces of wood, which are slotted to allow for height adjustment, and fit inside the bath forming a seat which is covered in rubber.
(d) 'Safa'-Bath seat.

86

Some parents, when bathing the severely handicapped child, have made a false bottom by using wooden slats made into a frame that can be placed in the bath, see fig. 63. The advantage is that the child can still lie in the water but the depth of the bath is considerably reduced. Always use very little water when bathing the more severely handicapped child so that he can be safely washed lying down, if he has some degree of head control one of the suction cushions made for the bath against which he can rest his head is useful. The more severely affected athetoid child may find sitting in the bath easier if supported by a broad band of webbing, see fig. 64.

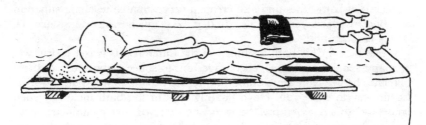

Figure 63. A frame formed of slats which is hooked over the sides of the bath.

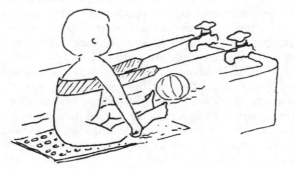

Figure 64. Webbing that may help the *athetoid* child to sit in the bath. A similar attachment can be used on the wash basin.

When the child becomes too heavy for you, try to lessen the strain on your back by sitting on a stool or kneeling on a cushion, by steadying yourself in this way you will be able to lift the child more easily.

We have already stressed the importance of accurate handling when lifting the child in and out of the bath. This of course, is even more important for the bigger child; refer again to chapter 11 on handling techniques. As we suggested for the younger child you may also find it helpful to wrap the child in a towel *before* lifting him out of the bath, first letting the water out.

If the child is to feel safe and enjoy his bath-time he must be handled slowly and be able to adjust himself while you move and wash him, the way to encourage his confidence is to tell him what you are going to do. Start off by touching and naming the taps, explain one is for hot water, the other for cold, show him how you turn the water on and off and demonstrate the difference in sound between a heavy or light flow of water, and let him feel the difference. Show him the plug and explain how it works, teach him to put it in and out, taking it around the tap when the water runs out, let him see you test the temperature of the water and explain to him why you do this. In this way you can make a game out of bath-times and also create a very valuable teaching situation and one in which you will also find it very much easier to secure the child's co-operation.

While he is in his bath let him feel the difference between a dry, wet or soapy sponge or flannel, encourage him to squeeze the water out, try to relate the way you are bathing him to the way he should bath his toys, let him try to copy you. Have floating toys in the bath including such household things as empty 'Squeezy' bottles, yoghurt containers, corks and so on and let him see, with you, the many ways in which these objects act in the water.

The cerebral palsied child can very often manage to play more easily with floating toys as he can move them around without undue effort. If the child enjoys the water use the opportunity, when possible, to repeat some of the games or movements that you have been teaching him during the day. If you have a spray attachment, use it as a method of increasing his awareness of various parts of his body, and if he can, ask him to name them. Rubbing him with a rough towel sometimes firmly, sometimes lightly, is a game for him and at the same time provides another learning situation. Adults often like to sing in their bath and if you find that your child likes to make a lot of noise as he splashes about in the water do encourage him, either by introducing new words, or if he is more advanced getting him to sing songs, nursery rhymes or games that incorporate actions with words.

Approach to independence in washing and bathing
Before starting to teach the child to wash himself it is worthwhile playing with him as suggested in chapter 17. The first lesson in learning to wash and dry his hands and face should start when he is either sitting using a basin of water placed on a table, or sitting in front of the washbasin, provided the basin is not too high, later standing in front of the basin, or on a box or chair in front of the basin. It should be remembered that to be completely independent the child has to be able to put in the plug, turn the taps on and off, pick up the soap and rub it either on his hands or on a flannel, and wash and dry his hands and replace his towel on the rail, take out the plug and wind the chain around the tap.

When the older child reaches the stage of bathing himself he may still be unable to get in and out of the bath, help him by giving him a box, a stool or a table of the right height on which he can stand or sit before stepping in. Make sure that he has something on which to hold, bars for this purpose can be purchased at most stores, see fig. 65. To begin with it is also important to see that the bath contains only a few inches of water.

We have tried to stress in this chapter, as we have in dealing with all everyday activities, the importance of working with your child towards independence. It is especially important that, in preparation for going to nursery school, your child should know how to wash and dry his own hands.

The following items of bathroom equipment will help the child when he reaches the stage of bathing himself:

A glove or mitt-type flannel;

A mitt-type loofah;

A wooden nail brush with dented sides which make it easier to grip, or a piece of webbing over the top of the brush through which the hand can be slipped.

A long-handled back brush;

A liquid soap container;

Soap and nail brush with suction caps to be placed against the bath, or on a bath tray;

Hand-spray attached to taps for rinsing, if a fixed spray is not a permanent attachment;

A large bath towel with a hole in the middle which can be slipped over the head, a terry-towelling wrap, or a towel with a tape on it which can be tied to the wall.

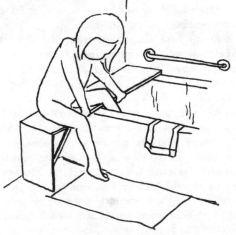

Figure 65. A simple way of making it easier for the child to get in and out of the bath and to manage on his own.

Chapter 8

DRESSING

The development stages that lead to the *normal* child's ability to dress and undress himself.

A *normal* child starts to co-operate with his dressing at about twelve months. He begins by holding out his foot for his shoe, or an arm for a sleeve.

At about eighteen months, at the same time as he achieves unsupported sitting and no longer has to rely on his hands for support, he will deliberately start to pull off his socks, shoes and hat. Previously he may have snatched them off, but unintentionally.

Between eighteen months and two years, he will co-operate more and more, starting to help to undress himself at about two years of age. He first starts to take off his clothes and gradually, as his hand movements become more co-ordinated, he begins to be able to put clothes on.

Between four and five, he can dress and undress except for buttons, ties and laces, and enjoys doing so; he attempts to lace his shoes but without appreciating whether or not the laces are in the correct holes. During this period he learns a lot by copying the way his mother does things and by experimenting with his own clothes or with those belonging to anyone else that he can find.

In dressing, as in all functional activities, the aim from the very beginning is to work towards maximum independence within the child's capabilities. The first stage in this programme is to gain the child's interest in what is being done, and as his abilities develop, to try to gain his co-operation.

It has to be remembered that a *normal* child is about twelve months old before he begins to co-operate, in a very simple way, with his dressing, and at least five or more years before he is completely independent. It takes him all this time before he can master the rather complicated movements required to put on and take off his clothes and to have sufficient balance to do this safely without falling over. A child of three-and-a-half should be able to lace the holes of his shoes, but until he is five or more will not be able to appreciate which holes to lace and in which direction. Similarly a child may push his feet into his shoes at three-and-a-half to four, but it does not become apparent to him which shoe goes on which foot until some time later. In fact the apparently simple activity of putting on and taking off one's clothes is far more complicated than is generally realised and follows a definite pattern of development, although with individual variations.

Dressing and undressing a cerebral palsied child

When dressing any young child the first thing we must do is to see that his clothes are within easy reach; with the handicapped child, whose handling is an added problem, this must always be our first priority, a clothes horse or back of a chair may be found useful for this purpose.

When a spastic child reaches the age of about eight or nine months, or earlier in some cases, one may begin to feel resistance to certain movements as he is dressed and undressed; his legs may be difficult to part to put on his nappy; his arms difficult to straighten to pull them through his sleeves, and so on.

The athetoid child does not present the same difficulties as the spastic child. The mother may find that her child kicks persistently, but at this stage she can still manage to dress him while he is lying down. As he grows and she tries to dress him when he is sitting up, she will find him much harder to handle due to his lack of head and trunk control and, in some cases, to extensor spasticity which may have developed.

It is therefore, often a good idea to dress and undress a baby lying across your knees on his tummy. This position gives one a good opportunity of combining handling and treatment. As explained in chapter 11 page 140 the child is maximally flexed in this position, but lying across your knees the pressure on his tummy is minimal, see fig. 66.

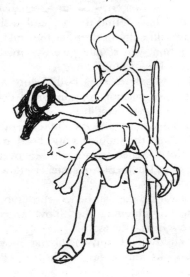

Figure 66. A good position to dress and undress a baby who has strong extensor spasms.

It is never a good idea to generalise in these cases, but most cerebral palsied children stiffen up and become more difficult to handle when they are lying on their backs, than when they are in any other position. This becomes more obvious as they grow older and athetosis and spasticity become stronger. Most children have a tendency, when in this position, to push the head and shoulders back, straightening and stiffening the hips and also the legs, which they often cross.

In order to gain the child's interest, he must first understand that he is going to be dressed and undressed, and what is being done and why. This is difficult if he is lying on his back and cannot see properly what is going on. If he is constantly dressed and undressed as if he were a doll, he cannot be blamed if he becomes quite detached and passive, showing no interest. Aim at dressing and undressing him, as soon as possible on his tummy, in side-lying or preferably sitting up, when he will be easier to manage and will have a better chance to see for himself what is going on and be stimulated to help whenever he can.

When a child is severely handicapped and is becoming heavier to handle, lying on his back is often the only possible way in which to dress and undress him. If you first put a hard pillow under his head, seeing that his shoulders are also raised a little, you will find it easier to bring his arms forward and to bend his hips and legs.

Lying on either side
With some garments it is not always practicable to dress a child while he is lying on his side, but it is suggested as an alternative because many mothers, to our knowledge, have found this a useful position as the child is not so stiff. If you have difficulty in dressing the child, and are unable to do so in a sitting position, you should give this method a trial. The following advantages have been found:

By rolling the child from side to side, both before and as you dress him, he is not in any one position for long, and does not therefore become so stiff and is easier to handle.

There is not so much tendency for the child to push himself back when he is on his side, and the shoulders and head are easier to bring forward. It is, therefore, easier to put clothes over the head and around the shoulders, and if there are fasteners down the back it is easier to reach them.

With the shoulder forward there will be less resistance to bringing the arm forward and to straightening the elbow, when, for example, putting his arms through his sleeves.

In many cases the child's legs and feet bend more easily in this position, and pants, socks and shoes can be put on with less of a struggle.

Being less stiff on his side, and with the improved head and eye-hand control which this position promotes, the child has a chance to see what is going on. He can start to co-operate and help with his dressing.

In certain cases mothers of babies with very stiff legs, have told us that they find side-lying an easier position to part the legs of the baby when putting on his nappy.

Sitting on your lap

It is most important to see that you have provided the child with an even safe base on which to sit, which means, among other things, not wearing a garment which has a slippery surface; if you are sitting on a high chair place a box under one or both feet, in this way giving yourself a more stable base. If the child is leaning backwards he will tend to fall back, if he takes his weight on one buttock only, his balance will become precarious and he may fall to one side, and you will start at a disadvantage when you try to dress him.

In many cases, the struggle one sometimes has to get a child's arm through his sleeve could have been avoided if it had been noticed that he had slipped back on his seat while being dressed, for it is very difficult to bring the arms forward while the trunk and shoulders remain back and the hips extended. A child who cannot sit and maintain his balance unsupported is easier to dress if he sits with his back to you leaning well forward, see figs. 67 a) b), in this position you can keep his legs apart and his hips bent. It is also an ideal position for the child who is inclined to straighten his hips and to fall back when one lifts his arms up or tries to bend his legs, especially when putting anything over his head.

When dressing or undressing the more severely handicapped child, sit in front of a mirror so that he can see what you are doing, this, of course, is merely a way of drawing his attention to what is going on. A mirror should *not* be used when he is ready to co-operate with his dressing, as obviously the reverse reflection in the mirror would only confuse him. When your child grows heavier and older, figs 68 a) b) show a position in which handling may be easier and which makes it possible for him to co-operate.

Advice which will help to overcome these difficulties

Always put clothes on the more affected arm or leg first.

Straighten the arm and then put the sleeve on; do not try to pull the child's arm through his sleeve if you feel resistance to straightening his elbow. *Never* take hold of his fingers and pull, this will immediately make the elbow bend.

If the child holds his head turned predominantly to one side, it will mean that the arm and leg towards which his face is turned will be harder for you to bend. At the same time the shoulder and hip on the other side will be apt to pull backwards and bend, making it difficult for you to straighten his arm, and the hand will probably be harder

93

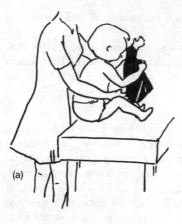
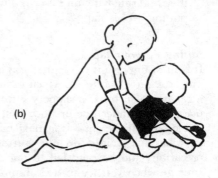

Figure 67
(a) and (b) By controlling the child from the back whether on the floor, or on a table or stool, you can keep his hips bent and his trunk well forward. In this way, lifting his head, lifting and bringing his arms forward, or lifting and bending his hips and legs will not immediately upset his balance. He is in a good position to see what you are doing and later to start co-operating with his dressing – and his hands will be in the same position as yours when he starts to dress himself.

to open. This, as we have explained earlier, can be avoided, to some extent, if you first see that he is sitting symmetrically.

If you have difficulty in getting the child's arm through the armhole or sleeve because he is pulling back at the shoulders, see that he is bending forward sufficiently at the hips, as this will make it easier to bring his arms forward.

If the child is inclined to fall forwards in sitting, the pressing down of his head and arms should be stopped *before* you start to dress him.

Always bend the child's leg before putting on socks and shoes, as with a straight leg the ankle and foot are stiffer and the toes more apt to turn under.

When putting on nappies have a pillow under the child's head or under his hips, this will make it easier to bend his hips and knees and to part them.

Suggestions for handling in dressing when the child starts to co-operate and finally takes over himself

Never miss an opportunity of encouraging the child to be independent, and immediately it is obvious that he *wants* to learn to try and help himself, encourage and praise him. At first an enormous amount of effort will be needed for very little achievement, in fact your patience will often run out before that of the child; do not be tempted to interfere unless of course he really gets into difficulties. Be sure that the task he has chosen is possible for him to achieve, for there is nothing more depressing for any of us than to tackle a difficult task with no reward at the end.

94

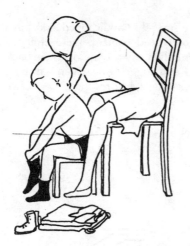

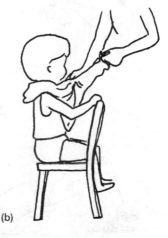

(a)

(b)

Figure 68
(a) Dressing the older heavier child, it is more satisfactory if you sit on a chair with your child on a stool in front of you with his feet flat on the floor.
(b) Sitting on a chair the child facing the back is a good position for dressing him; having a support directly in front of him which he can hold gives him confidence.

It is most important that the child should be as independent as possible by the time he reaches the age to go to nursery school, or later on, to school. You should therefore try to gain his help and interest at an early age, for the longer he is dressed and undressed by you the less inclined he will be to try for himself.

The child should be ready to start to dress and undress himself when he knows the parts of his body and is aware of himself in space, and can name or recognise his clothes, all helping him to relate his clothes to the parts of his body on which they go. He will also need to have sufficient balance to enable him to sit leaning forward freely, and to reach out with straight arms and grasp, maintaining his grasp regardless of the position of his arms, relying only occasionally on one arm for balance. The co-ordination and manipulative ability necessary to enable him to use his hands for dressing is described in chapter 16.

There are children who, though quite severely handicapped and have no sitting balance, nevertheless have good head control, these children can often start to dress and undress themselves when lying on their back or side, see figs. 69 for various positions and suggestions which will help such children to reach a degree of independence in dressing.

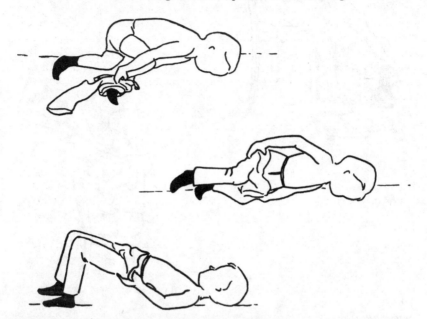

Figure 69. A child may have good head control, good arms and hands, but poor balance in sitting and therefore cannot dress and undress himself. You may find in side-lying he can do quite a lot for himself. In this position often the hips, legs and feet are easier to bend and he can keep his head and shoulders forward using his hands to grasp as shown. He must of course have quite a degree of mobility of his hips to dress in this position.

We have only to watch a *normal* baby being dressed and undressed to realise how a mother chatters spontaneously to him and how, even before he can talk, he babbles in response. Many cerebral palsied children are unable to respond in this way, and in time it may become easier for a mother not to bother to talk to her child and unfortunately to dress him in silence.

A *normal* child also has the advantage of being able to ask questions when he is puzzled; to learn by trial and error; to make use of and build up on previous experiences, and to ask for help immediately he requires it, yet it still takes about five years before *he* is almost independent. One must appreciate that the cerebral palsied child, with his many and varying difficulties, cannot be proficient in his dressing and undressing unless he is helped with all his problems.

As we dress the cerebral palsied child we can help him to get to know and to feel the various parts of his body by naming them as we do so. We should explain that his socks go on his feet and why; that his jersey goes over his head, and so on. We can point out the various openings in his clothes, relating clothes to the parts of the body, for example the head through the neck opening, and the arms through the sleeves. We can help him to relate such phrases as 'push your foot into your shoe', 'pull your arm out of your sleeve', as we perform the movement with him, and if he is beginning to talk, he should be asked to say the words at the same time as he does the actions. Later on colour can be included in the conversation, by comparing the colour of his clothes with other things around him. This can be followed, when he has reached the stage of understanding such things, by showing him which is the top and bottom, which is the right side and the left, which the inside and which the outside. In this way he will not only be learning how to dress himself but also accumulating knowledge which he can use in other activities.

It is therefore important, when finding out the difficulties the cerebral palsied child has when he starts to co-operate and take over his own dressing or undressing, that we try to understand all the problems involved, not merely those of manipulation. Your child's therapist will, of course, explain to you the specific problems with which he has to contend.

Parents should understand why, for example, a child is unable to put on his socks; perhaps he cannot distinguish the tops from the bottoms, or see the openings, or understand what is being asked of him. He may be unable to bend his hips sufficiently to enable him to bring his arms forward to reach his feet, or cannot bend one leg at a time, and his mother's attempts to bend his knee may result in his hips becoming straight, making him either fall backwards or, in some cases, collapse forwards. He may not be able to grasp when his arms are straight out in front of him, or to hold his socks and, at the same time, to pull them up, or he may drop the sock when he turns his head to look at his hand, or, common to many athetoid children, the grasping of one hand will often result in the opening of the other. His balance may not be secure enough in sitting, and he has to drop whatever he is holding to use one or both hands for support. These and many more problems may prevent him from putting on his socks – i.e. not one difficulty but a number of difficulties interacting on one another. Some of the more common problems the cerebral palsied child is faced with when he dresses himself are illustrated by figs. 70 a) to e)

When he starts to dress himself, watch carefully to see exactly how much he can manage on his own, and at which point he needs minimal help. The hemiplegic child will obviously use only his unaffected hand for dressing and this will cause stiffening in the affected hand, see figs. 71 a) to d). Do not *force* him to use his affected hand for dressing, see rather that he uses that arm and hand to support himself or as a 'holding' hand when necessary.

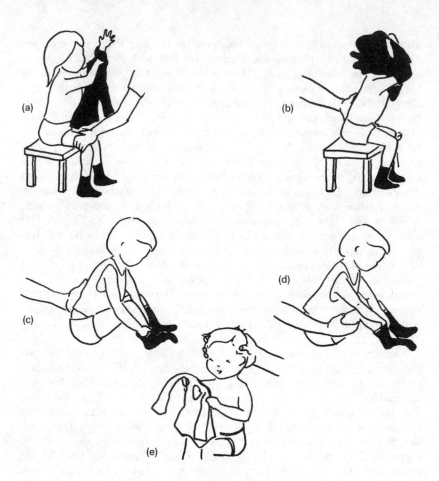

Figure 70. The sketches indicate the points of control with which to deal with the conditions described.

(a) The *athetoid* child when making an effort to speak, or as he raises his arms to dress, his feet may come off the floor and his legs may part. In this case apply pressure down over the knees keeping them together, or apply pressure on top of the feet.

(b) The *spastic* child when lifting his arms may extend his hips and knees and fall backwards. In this case, place your hand on the lower part of his spine and press him forward. With very *spastic* children keep the trunk well forward and at the same time hold the legs apart and outwards at the hips.

(c) and (d) Pulling socks up, one leg may straighten and he will fall back lifting his arms and losing his grasp. Placing your hand on the lower part of his spine will help to keep his hips and legs bent and enable him to keep his shoulders forward and use his hands. If his grasp is poor when his arm is straight, help by keeping the leg bent by holding under his thigh.

(e) Looking at their hands while they use them is difficult for many cerebral palsied children. Grasp shown gives good control of the head. Do *not* use this grip if it makes the child push back with his head.

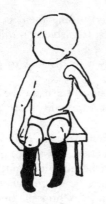

(a)

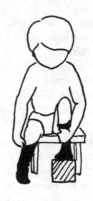

(b)

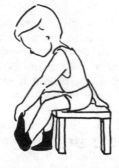

(c)

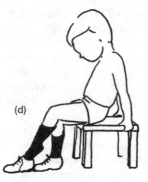

(d)

Figure 71
(a) Shows the difficulty the *hemiplegic* child has to pull off his socks, and the effect of using the good hand has on the affected arm and hand.
(b) By placing his affected leg on a box and bringing his arm forward, the child inhibits his own 'associated reactions'.
(c) and (d) Show ways requiring less effort to take off socks and shoes. The child should sit on a box or stool so that his feet are flat on the floor.

Physical difficulties experienced by the child when dressing and undressing himself

Difficulty in looking at what he is doing.

Insufficient balance when he starts to use both hands; often the result of 'associated reactions', i.e. movements of the arms and hands making the legs stiff and the hips to straighten, or in the case of the athetoid child, causing his feet to lift off the ground and him to lose his balance.

Poor co-ordination between the two hands and insufficient fine co-ordination of the fingers.

Trying to hold with one hand while he moves the other.

Inability to grasp, regardless of the position of the arm.

99

Having to hold and lift his clothes, especially pulling them over his head, without falling back; opening his clothes, for which he will need both hands.

Starting to put on his sock and reaching down to his foot to pull it over the heel.

Starting to pull down his pants; putting the second arm in the sleeve of his coat; doing up and undoing fasteners, especially those at the back.

These are general points of advice and obviously they may need adapting to meet the specific difficulties of each child. *Do not* continue to dress and undress your child from habit or just because it is quicker. If he is ever to learn to be independent, he must first be taught what to do and how to do it, and then be encouraged to try for himself, first with guidance and then on his own. Figs 72 to 76 illustrate various positions which will make it easier for the child when he starts to dress himself, and later to manage on his own.

Finally, but very important, the child must be given a chance to manage on his own, remember that he will learn to undress himself before he will learn to dress. This has the advantage that undressing is usually done in the evening when there is less rush and one can be more patient. If pressure on your time is a problem the week-end is often a good time to allow the child to experiment. Leave him alone one day, when you think that he should be doing more for himself, while you carry on with your work, and on your return you may be surprised to find what his capabilities really are. Children can be very crafty; we have known cases where a mother has been called to the front door or the telephone to find on her return, that her often bored and apparently helpless child has dressed himself, something which up to that moment no one believed he could possibly do.

Clothes

Children enjoy being told how nice they look; cerebral palsied children are no exception and should be encouraged to take a pride in their appearance. When old enough, and within reasonable limits, they should be allowed to help to choose their clothes and decide what they would like to wear. Fortunately the designs of children's clothes these days are quite suitable for many handicapped children, therefore adaptations can be kept to a minimum.

All mothers, no doubt through trial and error, will have bought or made types of clothes most suitable for easing the task of dressing and undressing their child; washing and ironing is time-consuming and I am sure that you have all found that dark and patterned materials do not show up stains as clearly as light colours. It is advisable to choose stain-repellent materials and those that are non-shrinkable and need little ironing.

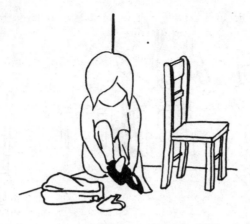

Figure 72. Where balance in sitting is still not good enough to allow the child to have both hands free to dress himself and he has the tendency to fall backwards, use the corner of the wall to give him support. See that his clothes are within reach by his side, and if necessary have a stool or chair for him to hold.

(a)

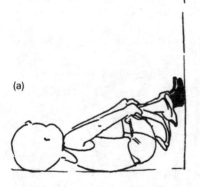

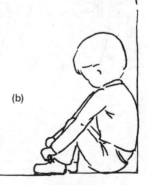

(b)

Figure 73. Two ways of making use of a wall.
(a) By pressing his feet against the wall the child is able to lift his hips while he pulls up his trousers. This is a good position for the *athetoid* child as it provides him with the necessary stability.
(b) Supporting himself against the wall the *spastic* child can keep his legs bent as he leans forward to do up his shoes.

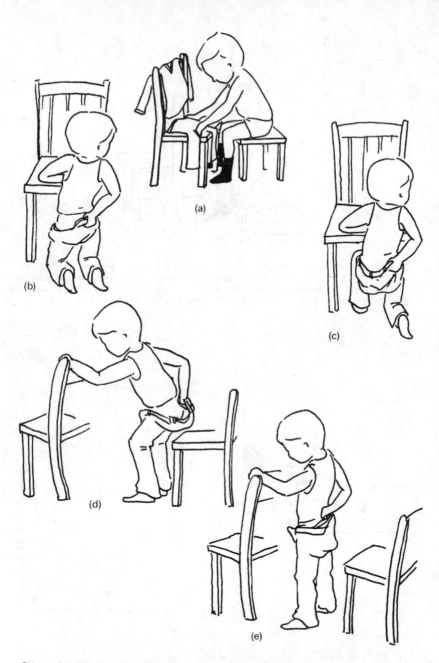

Figure 74. These five drawings indicate the positions in which the child gains confidence when he starts to dress and undress himself. Place a chair or table in front of him so that he can use it for support when necessary; place his clothes out for him to begin with.

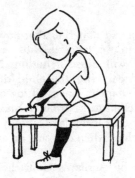

Figure 75. By turning sideways when sitting on a box or stool, the *spastic* child may find it easier to bend one leg without straightening the other and to reach his foot. Balance also will be better in this position.

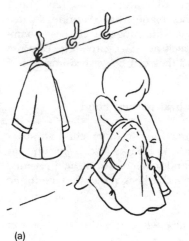

(a)

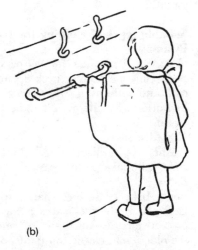

(b)

Figure 76. Dressing and undressing means being able to cope with outdoor clothes, and when starting nursery school hanging them up.
(a) Kneeling on their knees gives some children a wider and firmer base than when standing and helps them to pull their coat off without over-balancing.
(b) A bathroom rail provides a useful rail for the child to hold onto when taking off a cape or coat.

103

Materials

Other than for linings, avoid materials that have a slippery surface, such as nylon; be careful not to use materials with a rough surface for use next to the skin as rubbing will cause irritation. Nylon material not only makes picking up and carrying the child difficult but, as we have mentioned in an earlier chapter, makes sitting on a chair with a slippery surface difficult for the child to keep his balance. You may have noticed when your own dress or coat is made of a shiny material that it is harder for you to handle your child when carrying or having him sitting on your lap.

Knitted clothes made of 'Acrilan', 'Courtelle' or 'Orlon' are always a good buy as they keep their shape and colour when washed, and as they have plenty of 'give' they are easiest to take on and off. If you decide to knit or crochet a cape or poncho, a wool and 'Courtelle' mixture can be recommended. 'Terylene', 'Bri-nylon', 'Dacron' or 'Crimplene' are excellent materials as they are easy to iron and withstand considerable wear and tear.

Since my first edition many parents of children who have poor circulation, have spoken highly of clothes made from thermo-insulated materials, this material is now used in a wide range of clothes. Foam-backed materials used in outer clothes such as coats, capes etc. can also be recommended as good 'insulators' and they can be washed and ironed quickly.

Suitable types of clothing for the cerebral palsied child
Pyjamas

'All in one' pyjamas for young children; for the older child slip-over blouse top, elastic type neck opening with no buttons, elastic around the cuffs and bottoms of pyjama legs. Tops and trousers can be held together by buttons; for the more handicapped child a back panel may be found useful.

Nightdresses

Elastic type neck opening – back opening with tapes for the younger child will make potting easier.

Pants

For a baby or severely handicapped young child, press studs, zips or lacing at both sides saves a lot of lifting; it is now possible to buy protective pants which are soft and serviceable and tie at both sides. For the older child elastic top pants, or pants with a dropped front attached to the waistband with 'Velcro' should be used.

Vests

The most suitable are those which have the largest openings for the head. The 'envelope cross-over' opening for the younger child, and for the older child a 'scoopneck' with shoulder straps. Where a wide shoulder strap is preferred the seam can, if you wish, be opened and tape used, 'Velcro' fastening, or loop and button be sewn on to make it easier for the child.

Parents report favourably on 'Thermotactyl' vests, when used for children who feel the cold.

Socks

Good fitting socks are as important as good fitting shoes and are one item of clothing that should not be passed down through the family. If your child is wearing short trousers, knee-length knitted socks are the most suitable. While socks are comparatively easy for a child to take off, putting them on can present quite a problem, tubular socks with no heel shaping are a good type of sock until he becomes more proficient.

Tights

For young children choose the tights that come right up with a bib-front and fasten at the shoulders, i.e. using the same front as for dungarees. For children starting to crawl tights can be reinforced with squares of leather or fabric material.

Sleeves

All sleeves should be as loose as possible. The raglan or dolman sleeve provides the largest opening for the arm; this type of sleeve is available in a variety of garments. It is equally important to have an opening at the bottom of the sleeve, large enough through which to slip your fingers and pull the child's *hand* through. In some cases opening the seam from the neck down the arm will make it easier to get the head through, and where there is a tight cuff the under seam can be opened. Open seams can be edged with 'Velcro'.

Shirts

One of the difficulties with shirts is to keep them tucked into the trousers. This can be remedied by buttoning them onto the trousers or pants, or by means of tapes sewn to the bottom of the shirt. For the older child who has to wear long-sleeved shirts which need buttons at the cuff use two buttons connected by elastic, or buttons sewn together with a long shank. To save buttoning and unbuttoning, edge each side of the opening of the front of the shirt with 'Velcro' sew up the button-holes or sew on extra large press studs.

Jerseys

The most important point with jerseys is to see that there is an easy opening for the head; often they have elastic woven into the material around the neck. Jerseys can be v-necked, polo-necked or scoop-necked.

Dresses

The shift or pinafore dress is the most practicable, being simple to put on and needing no fastenings. Some designs have buttons on the shoulders and these can be replaced with 'Velcro' if you wish. You may find it easier to dress your child if you buy the type of pinafore dress that has buttons both on the shoulders and down one side. Shifts and pinafore dresses can be made in a variety of materials and are also easy to knit; a t-shirt, blouse or jersey can be worn underneath. For the more severely handicapped older child, a dress will be easier to put on if a zip-fastener is put down the back so that both arms can be put through the sleeves first. Many parents who have tried 'Bibette' dresses with the interchangeable fronts made of repellent cotton or 'P.V.C.' have found them useful; parents who make dresses often use this design.

Trousers

Trousers with elasticated tops are obviously the most practicable as they do not require fastenings around the waist. When your child gets older replace fly buttons either with a 'Velcro' strip or a zip-fastener. For young boys, still in nappies, short trousers for indoors make handling easier. Dungarees in combination with a t-shirt or jersey are recommended for the child who is starting to crawl and move around the house, patches of carpet provide extra protection for the knees. It is now possible to buy 'Velbex' dungarees that can be sponged clean. Stretch-flared trousers now in fashion, even for very young children, save having to open the inside or outside seam to make it easier to get them on or off.

Shoes

Before discussing the various types of shoes recommended for the cerebral palsied child, let us consider some of the problems. The cerebral palsied child having poor balance is often 'late' in standing. In some cases he has the added problem of spasticity which normally results in him having 'immobile' feet, the weight being taken on the inner-side of the foot with the toes often clawing, or bunched and pulled together in a sideways direction. Other children have the problem of athetosis or general low-tone which results in unstable feet – the weight taken on the outer or inner side of the foot. In the hemiplegic child the good foot shows exaggerated balance reactions – seen as excessive movements – the affected foot being inactive.

To illustrate the important part the feet play in our balance try this experiment yourself. Stand on one leg and feel the amount of movement in your foot and toes. Now stand with your weight on the inner sides of your foot and try to balance on one leg – you will find that it is impossible. Claw your toes and get someone to push you, and you will immediately fall forwards and lose your balance. Walk with your weight first on the inner, then on the outer edges of your feet, and see the effect on your whole walking pattern and general posture of your body.

These are some of the problems your child may have when trying to walk, you will now have realised that without a good fitting and supportive basic shoe that can be adapted when necessary, your child's feet would not only become more immobile resulting in poor balance, but that his standing and walking could only deteriorate. We have only to think of the discomfort and poor walking that results when we have badly fitting shoes.

Advice on shoes must inevitably be generalised but here are a few pointers; – the first pair of shoes are just as important or even more important than subsequent pairs. When the child is able to walk on his own, take him with you to the shoe-shop and watch him walking in the shoes before deciding to buy. Be sure to know his correct size, possibly

106

there is a difference between his left and right foot, this may be the result, for example, of taking more weight on one foot than the other – most of us do in fact have one foot larger than the other. The Spastics Society publish a list called 'Odd Shoes' giving the names of the firms that provide this service.

See that his shoes are easy to put on and take off, and that he can get his heel down and his toes well into them, a shoe that opens down the front will make this easier.

If your child is starting to put on and take off his own shoes see that there are no unnecessary buckles, difficult laces etc. and satisfy yourself, whilst in the shop, that he can manage them himself. Elastic sided shoes, elastic laces and eyelets that can be adapted to make lacing easier are now available. A narrow heeled shoe is not recommended, i.e. the type of shoe which has a continuous piece of leather stretching from the top of the back of the shoe to the sole and has no heel, this type of shoe does *not* give adequate support.

While some young children are proud of their shoes and will even demand to keep them on in bed, there are those who continually take their shoes off, the makers of 'Remploy Bootees' have designed bootees which make this much harder for the child to do.

Children in general, and handicapped children in particular, are very hard on their shoes. In England 'North Hill Plastics Ltd' make an excellent colourless plastic for protecting shoes, so immediately the shoes show signs of wear ask your therapist to reinforce the toe caps, or advise you where you can get this done, do not wait until a hole appears. Many mothers, as an added precaution, have this material put on a new pair of shoes *before* they are worn. New products for reinforcing shoes are frequently being introduced – so watch for them; experiments are being made to mould plastic toe-caps onto children's shoes, but at present these are not commercially produced.

It may, of course, be necessary for your child to have a special pair of boots or shoes prescribed, or an additional support provided to build the shoe up on the inner or outer side, or for alterations to be made to the heel. Sometimes platform soles are recommended, or in the case of toes that continually claw, a 'raise' in a sandal may be necessary. Whatever alterations are made to the shoes it is essential to watch your child carefully for the first two or three weeks of use so that any change can be made without delay. Your child may not be able to tell you that his shoes are uncomfortable, so look carefully to see if he has any pressure sores on his feet and look at the soles and heels to see if they are being worn evenly.

For older children who can walk on their own, parents often find that their child will walk better in such as 'baseball boots', varying types of sandals, including for mildly affected hemiplegic children 'Scholls' or 'Clarks' sandals, and even sports-training shoes which are soft with padded tongues and arch support. The choice of such shoes by a child, may be the result of seeing his friends wearing them, however if they improve his walking, and he will certainly be keen to show you that it does, there is no harm in letting him try.

If wellingtons are worn do see that these fit well and if not, that the child wears a bootee or extra thick pair of socks, wellingtons in 'P.V.C.' with either short or long legs are made with a warm lining. For the severely handicapped older child who cannot keep his shoes on, a soft leather sole can be sewn to a knitted sock or tights.

For nearly all young children we recommend as their first pair of shoes 'Shoo Shoos' – available only in white, sizes 2 – 7, 'Remploy Bootees' – available in white, brown or black, sizes 2 – 13. In England 'Remploy Bootees' can be obtained through a M.O.H. prescription. Figs. 77 a) b) c) illustrate some of the shoes and boots to which we have referred.

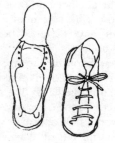
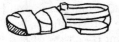
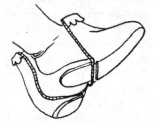
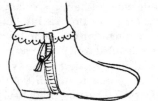

(a)

(b)

(c)

Figure 77

(a) 'Remploy Bootee' similar in design to 'Shoo-Shoos' – for details see list of suppliers.

(b) Sandal showing 'raise' to help inhibit clawing of toes, especially useful in the case of the *hemiplegic* child; a platform sole may also be found beneficial in some cases.

(c) Boots with a zip side-opening making it easier for the child to put on and take off his own boots.

Overalls

'P.V.C.', 'Velbex' and allied materials are best for overalls as they can be washed down without being taken off; if overalls are used at mealtimes be sure that they are the type with deep pockets around the hem, to catch falling pieces of food, back fasteners will be found most satisfactory. When you are joining in messy play with your child, or at feeding times, it is advisable for you also to wear an apron or overall of 'P.V.C.' or similar material.

Bibs

Absorbent terry-towelling bibs with waterproof backing and ties at the waist, or bibs which are backed with absorbent filling provide the best protection for young children. Some mothers, of children who dribble constantly, find that a piece of terry-towelling placed under the child's dress or top helps to absorb excessive moisture. For the older child the long-life 'Dikky' bib made of non-toxic soft polythene with a specially shaped pocket is recommended as it is so easy to wipe down.

Coats and Hats

Cloaks, capes and ponchos are now popular and are designed even for very small children, having no sleeves they are much simpler for parents and later for the child himself to manage, if required a loop of elastic can be inserted for the shoulder, and one for the arm to prevent them slipping off. In particular, the design of the poncho is so simple that it can easily be made up in any material, knitted or even crocheted. A removable hood attached to cloaks and capes is useful for the winter. Quilted anoraks and foam-backed coats are often difficult to put on and take off, therefore it is important to see that they are large enough when you buy them. For added warmth under a coat, a simple idea is to knit, or make in warm material, a sleeveless coat or waistcoat which will be warm but not bulky, and is easy to put on and take off. For a baby a sleeping bag can be a good substitute for a coat. Macintoshes with combined hoods are also made in a cape design and are recommended.

Gloves

Mittens are sometimes easier to get on than gloves, especially for the hemiplegic child; to prevent losing attach a piece of elastic or tape for the wrist.

Hats

These are often difficult to keep on – the hood type with band under the chin and snap-fastener, or combined hood and scarf are the most serviceable.

Fastenings

The most difficult part of dressing or undressing for any child is the fastenings, while it might be quite simple for him to open and close fastenings on clothes laid out in front of him for practise, it is quite a different matter when the fasteners are on the clothes he is wearing; it is not so easy for him to look at what he is doing, and the manipulation and co-ordination of using both hands becomes more difficult. Try out different types of fastenings with your child, and then you can decide if a zip-fastener with a ring, ball or tape, shank buttons, large press studs, or even sewing up some button-holes and sewing a strip of 'Velcro' underneath, is the answer. Your aim is independence and it is worthwhile taking extra time and trouble choosing fasteners that the child can manage.

Clothes for Babies

When choosing clothes for babies and young children these days, we are no longer faced with the problem of finding suitable materials, as most manufacturers use materials that are easily washed, keep their colour and are non-shrinking, many of them stain-resistant. Clothes are designed to make dressing and nappy changing as simple as possible. A few garments that our mothers have found satisfactory for young babies are the wrap-over styled vests with tie fastenings, followed by vests with envelope shaped neck opening. 'Mothercare' polucho cotton-vincel pants and vest, and their 'Baby Stretch' garments made from cotton-'Bri-nylon' stretch-terry which include their 'all-in-one' garments, jumper with envelope neck, two-piece playsuits and 'Baby's First Pull Ups'.

Chapter 9

FEEDING

by Helen Mueller

Miss Mueller, speech therapist, spent five years in Zurich teaching speech-handicapped children and training student teachers; then four years in the USA and ten years teaching at the University of Zurich and Friborg and at the University Childrens Clinics in Berne, Munich, Innsbruck and Vienna; she has held a post as Consultant Speech Therapist in Germany and Austria. Miss Mueller has lectured and taught in many parts of Europe and in the USA on pre-speech and the associated problems of feeding.

From birth and through the early years, feeding presents problems for most cerebral palsied children. We, however, need hardly stress the importance of proper food intake for the child's physical, emotional, social and dental development. A good feeding pattern is an essential for future speech.

STAGES OF NORMAL DEVELOPMENT
The following outlines the stages of development of feeding of a *normal* child and enables comparison to be made with those experienced by the cerebral palsied child.

During the first few months a baby takes food in by what is known as a 'sucking-swallowing reflex'.

As this reflex is insufficient from birth in some cerebral palsied babies, mealtimes can present real difficulties for him and for his mother, either because he will become impatient and tense and start crying or else he escapes by falling asleep for most, if not all the feeding time; sometimes the mother will then enlarge the hole in the nipple, tilt the baby back and let the liquid trickle down. This is passive feeding and whilst it may help to get the food down, it usually causes choking and certainly does nothing to help to develop better mouth functioning.

After the first few weeks, the mother starts to give the *normal* baby juice with a small spoon and he will suck the liquid in; after about six months and when he begins to sit, he is ready to learn to take the liquid or food from a spoon with his lips and transfer it for swallowing, a process which generally takes about a month or more before he is proficient.

During this time the cerebral palsied baby may appear also to be

111

sucking by opening and closing motions of his mouth but his attempts are ineffectual, so once again the liquid food has to be poured down the back of his throat. If you offer him semi-solid liquids, such as yoghurt, he is very likely to manage earlier and more easily to swallow it taking it with his lips.

At six to seven months the *normal* baby begins to munch, in effect he is getting ready to be able to bite off and to chew solids; gagging occurs much less frequently now and dribbling will generally be noticed only during the teething period. These are signs that oral control is developing. The cerebral palsied child is often unable to chew and instead makes forward motions with his tongue, pushing the food back out or glueing it to the roof of his mouth; the food may get squashed but it is not chewed and when it reaches the back of the mouth it is uncontrolled, generally leading to gagging and choking.

About one month after a *normal* baby has learned to take food from a spoon, he will, whilst in a sitting position, be ready to drink liquids from a cup or a glass. In the early stage there is bound to be some inco-ordination resulting in the liquids leaking out onto the side of the mouth together with some coughing and gulping; these effects will continue to be seen until his oral control has become efficient enough to enable him to deal adequately even with wholly liquid foods. The cerebral palsied child, however, will probably be unable to get his lips 'attached' to the cup or glass whilst his tongue will very likely protrude over or under the rim of the cup or glass; you may already have noticed these abnormalities while he was having his bottle. The mouth making the same unsuccessful opening and closing motions, the tongue pushing forward as the child tries to drink. These abnormalities are similar to those described when we were speaking of chewing; this results once again in the child's head having to be tilted backwards letting the liquid run in and down passively which provokes choking, coughing and air-gulping.

As drinking through a straw usually calls for good oral control the use of straws for drinking by a *normal* child is usually not attempted until he is three or four years old. The type of sucking used when drinking through a straw requires much finer co-ordination of the lips than is necessary for reflex sucking by the infant. Drinking through straws is something the cerebral palsied child can seldom manage as instead of holding the straw and sucking it with his lips, he puts the straw into his mouth like a nipple and bites it or holds it up so that the liquid flows in passively. This lack of co-ordination will show itself by the irregular flow and by coughing, choking and air-gulping.

FEEDING AND THE CEREBRAL PALSIED CHILD

What are the major feeding problems of the cerebral palsied child? They are lack of mouth, head and trunk control, lack of sitting balance, and inability to bend his hips sufficiently to enable him to stretch his arms forward to grasp and to maintain that grasp irrespective of the position of his arms; finally his inability to bring his hands to his mouth and his lack of eye-hand co-ordination.

It must be stressed that it is only by careful observation and analysis of the child's disabilities and abilities can we hope to help him. We must not expect improvement in the child's feeding abilities until we have helped him to acquire the fundamental abilities which will make self-feeding possible – that is the ability to move his head, jaw, lips and tongue independently from the body and hands while having good sitting balance.

Some positions for feeding

We continue to stress that adequate control of the 'whole' child is essential while he is being fed. Unless this control is secured he will become more spastic or will have increased involuntary movements, even before the bottle or spoon is placed in his mouth, thus making it harder for him to suck or to use his lips; whenever possible do avoid placing your hand on the back of the child's head for support as this will immediately cause him to push back.

A good feeding position for the young infant and the severely handicapped baby is shown in fig. 78 (a)(b)(c). The baby's legs are kept apart and scissoring is made impossible by your body, his arms and head are brought forward from the shoulders, and kept in this position by placing your hand flat and with pressure on his lower chest, see figs. 79 (a)(b). If you need that hand for jaw-control use your forearm to apply pressure on the child's chest. Have his food at your side so that the child can see it and not on the table where he would have to stretch backwards to find out where each spoonful is coming from. This is a position which allows good overall control as well as good eye-contact and is especially useful for those children who have a tendency towards asymmetry; by sitting closer to the table and placing the wedge at a steeper angle see fig. 80(a)(b) you will gradually be able to get the child into a more upright position.

A good feeding position for the baby who has some sitting balance is on your lap, controlling him as shown in fig. 81. You can keep him from throwing himself into extension by flexing his hips and placing your leg under his knees higher than the leg under his buttocks. When a child needs extra support for his lower back or his shoulder, while at the same time jaw control is necessary, you may find your arm becoming over-tired; to avoid this rest the elbow of the arm you are using to support your child on the table and cushion it with a pillow. As stated previously it is very important to place the food in front of the child and not behind.

As soon as the child has developed some head and trunk control, feed him whilst he is sitting on a chair – do not prolong unnecessarily feeding him on your lap. Make sure that when the child is sitting on a chair beside or opposite you that you are on a level with him or even a little lower than he is, otherwise the tendency will be for him to have to look up to you and push back his head.

Be careful to see that the child does not sit with a rounded back or he will compensate by lifting his chin, making swallowing almost impossible. Have *you* ever tried to swallow with your head tilted back? See also that his hips and knees are at a right angle and his legs are slightly apart; groin straps will occasionally be necessary to maintain this position.

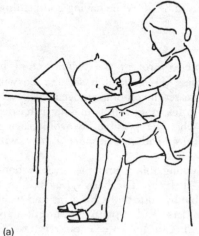

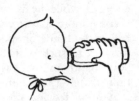

(a)

(b)

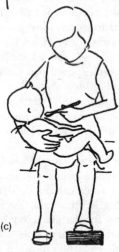

(c)

Figure 78
(a) Bottlefeeding. When needed, mother applies pressure to the chest with a flat hand and jaw control during sucking.
(b) The baby puts his hands around the bottle.
(c) *Right.* Feeding of a baby in half-sitting position with head and both arms forward.

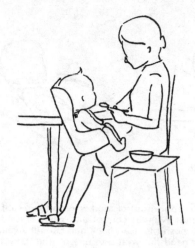

(a)

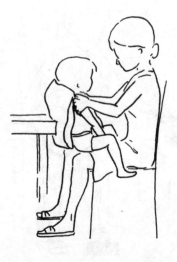

(b)

Figure 79
(a) Half-sitting position for the child with some sitting balance. Remember to put the food in front of him. If the child still needs support, an 'Infant Seat' can be used resting against the table edge.
(b) When sitting balance improves, sit the baby up straight with his legs abducted and his hips well flexed. You may still have to control him from the shoulders.

115

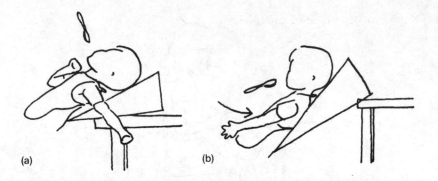

(a)   (b)

Figure 80
(a) *Wrong*. The baby is placed in front of mother on a foam-rubber wedge, which rests against the table-edge. Without control and when the spoon is presented from above, the baby will push his head back and cannot swallow properly.
(b) *Right*. If you put your hand flat with pressure on the baby's lower chest and present the spoon from the front, you help him to control his head and to swallow.

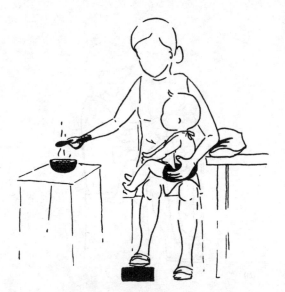

Figure 81. When feeding the baby in a sitting position on your lap, you can prevent hyperextension by putting your leg under his knees on a stool to give him more hip flexion. If he needs support on his lower back or shoulders, put your arm on a pillow on the table. The food must be in front of the child.

116

Controlling Mouth Functioning

Besides controlling the 'whole' child during feeding we can apply additional control in the oral area which will help to improve his sucking-swallowing reflex and his ability both to eat from a spoon, and drink from a cup.

When control of the muscles of the mouth is lacking, it is necessary to apply oral control to improve feeding. This is applied with two fingers: middle finger and index if applied from the side fig. 82(a) or middle finger and thumb if applied from the front fig. 82(b). The child will probably respond on the first occasion to oral control by pushing against it, but give him time to adjust; do not pull his head back but keep it straight with his neck slightly stretched and you will soon find that he accepts this help.

Before presenting the bottle, spoon or cup to the child, apply oral control, otherwise you will find that his efforts to reach them or to open his mouth to receive them will often result in hyper-extension of the whole body.

With the gradual improvement of oral functioning you will gradually be able to lessen and finally withdraw oral control.

The most common of all problems that make feeding of the cerebral palsied child so difficult are tongue-thrust, prolonged and exaggerated bite reflex, abnormally strong gag reflex, tactile hypersensitivity in the oral area and dribbling. Good oral control is therefore a most important factor for children with oral disfunction.

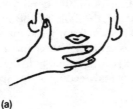

(a)

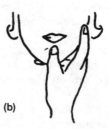

(b)

Figure 82
(a) Oral control as applied when the child is on your right side with your arm around his head: index finger between chin and lower lip, middle finger behind chin applying constant firm pressure.
(b) Oral control as applied from the front: thumb between chin and lower lip, middle finger applied firmly just behind the chin.

Hypersensitivity

Touch in the mouth will increase sensitivity and become exaggerated if there is over-stimulation by the use of a nipple, spoon, straw or teat or if a mother wipes a dribbling child's wet mouth and chin often during feeding and at other times during the day. Guard against hypersensitivity by avoiding such over-activity and where possible make use of jaw-control. Where hypersensitivity has become very pronounced consult your speech therapist.

Dribbling and Open Mouth

This is a common problem amongst cerebral palsied children and will certainly not disappear when parents continue merely to remind the children throughout the day to close their mouths and to swallow. The obedient child will of course try to draw in the saliva but lacking the ability to swallow properly, his efforts will be of momentary effect only and the accumulated saliva will dribble out again just as soon as he re-opens his mouth with an extensor spasm, when feeding, babbling or trying to speak. You will help your child more if occasionally during the day you place your finger across between his upper lip and nose, exercising firm and continuous pressure and do this without talking to him or interrupting his play; gradually you will find that spontaneous mouth-closure and spontaneous swallowing will take place. In addition continue to use jaw-control in feeding and drinking as this will establish a proper swallowing pattern.

Bottle-drinking

With babies who have an abnormal sucking-swallowing reflex, improvement can immediately be achieved by combined body, head and jaw-control. The old-fashioned round nipple is the easiest for the cerebral palsied infant. If he still has difficulties in sealing his lips around the nipple, bring his cheeks forward with two fingers of the hand you are using for jaw-control and, if you have enlarged the hole in the nipple, thicken the formula of the liquid which will stop it from trickling down into his throat uncontrolledly. If the child is so severely handicapped that he has no sucking-swallowing reflex and needs to be tube-fed, the only way to get him off the tube and to more normal feeding is by spoon-feeding.

Spoon-feeding

Here again jaw-control is very important but often will not be sufficient to enable the cerebral palsied baby to start taking semi-solid foods from a spoon; here firm pressure with the spoon flat on his tongue will prevent the tongue from pushing forward and bring about spontaneous use of lips and tongue. In these cases, use a metal or bone spoon, as a plastic spoon will break very easily and is generally too deep, see fig. 83 (a). Make sure that the spoon is not too deep otherwise the food cannot

118

easily be scraped out of it with the lips, or one too long and pointed which might cause stimulation of the gag reflex see fig. 83 (b). The spoon should *always* be presented and placed *from midline, never* from the side when feeding any type of cerebral palsied child.

Having pressed the spoon on the tongue firmly be sure to take it out without scraping it on the upper teeth or lip, see figs. 84 (a)(b) at the same time do let the child try to get the food off with his upper lip while you press with the spoon on his tongue. Feeding will be easier for him if, to begin with, you place only a small amount of food in the front of the spoon. As soon as you withdraw the spoon see that the mouth is closed so as to keep the tongue inside for carrying the food around the mouth instead of letting the tongue push the food out.

If spoon feeding presents real difficulty, as a last resort use your fingers but then only with such solids as meat, bread, fruit etc.

When introducing spoon-feeding you will find that strained but fairly dry food is best to begin with, liquids and thinly strained foods are considerably more difficult and those of a mixed texture such as thin vegetable soup will always remain the most difficult with which to cope.

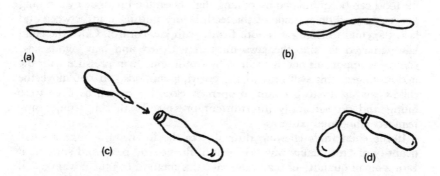

Figure 83
(a) *Wrong*. The spoon is too deep and pointed.
(b) *Right*. The spoon should be fairly flat and rounded.
(c) To adapt the metal spoonhandle it can be cut to a point and pushed firmly into a tool handle.
(d) To adapt the metal spoon, bend it at the necessary angle to get it straight into the mouth.

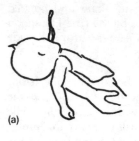

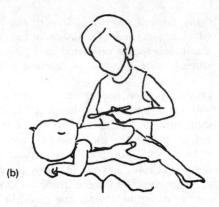

(a)

(b)

Figure 84
(a) *Wrong*. The child is fed while he is totally passive in hyperextension, food is scraped off on the upper teeth, causing gagging, coughing and choking.
(b) The child can never develop good swallowing in hyperextension with one arm behind mother.

Chewing

To develop chewing it is best to place such food as particles of meat or crusts of brown bread by hand between his teeth on the side of his mouth, helping him to close his mouth by using jaw-control, biting off the food can be stimulated by pulling slightly on the bread or by scraping the crusty food on the side of the teeth before putting it in between and help the child to close his mouth firmly with jaw-control. Once the child has managed to bite, the jaws must stay closed and here again jaw-control is important and is secured by continuous firm pressure with the middle finger; this will lead to the chewing motions; do not move the child's jaw or try to get him to open or close his mouth as if he were biting and do *not* apply intermittent pressure – all this would only reinforce abnormal patterns.

If the child finds chewing difficult, try the following – take a small quantity of best quality raw beef, cut a 'finger-size' piece and sprinkle it with a small quantity of seasoning salt; this method has the advantage of being absolutely safe as a piece cannot be bitten off with the danger of it slipping back into the child's throat. While you hold onto one end of it, the child, with jaw-control, chews on the other end and whilst he is doing so chews out the nourishing juices of the meat and at the same time is practising swallowing and after a while he can start on the unchewed end of the finger of meat. It is much better to practise this at the beginning of the main meal as it is an effective preparation for chewing.

If during feeding a piece of food slips back into the child's throat and gets stuck, make sure to bring him well forward into good flexion at once and do not become nervous; if you react quickly and calmly there will be no danger, as the piece will come back out and the child will not be unduly frightened. *Do not* pat his back as this causes inhalation and may lead to aspiration.

Drinking

It is difficult for the small child with oral disfunction to learn to drink liquids and help will be necessary for some time; here again careful control of the whole body, the head and of the jaw, in particular, is of the utmost importance, see figs. 85 (a)(b). As we have already said, it is by no means enough merely to get the liquid down by some means or another, as then the child is forced into a totally passive role and will not learn, and you will be in an even worse situation than before as oral-hypersensitivity is likely to increase, and with it choking and gagging.

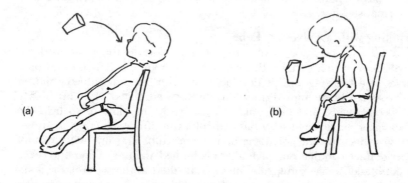

(a)   (b)

Figure 85
(a) *Wrong*. The cup is presented from above and the child is tilted back.
(b) *Right*. The child is in a sitting position for drinking, with the trunk and head well forward, the beaker is presented from the front.

Start by using a plastic beaker and one with a projecting rim, see fig. 86(a), cut out an opening on one side for the nose, see fig. 86(b) this will enable you to tilt the beaker until the last drops have gone and avoids the necessity of bending the child's head back, see fig. 86(c), also you will be able to see and control what is happening at his mouth.

The most important single factor in learning to drink is the mouth closure, as it is only if the jaws remain closed and the rim of the beaker is resting between the child's lips, will he eventually be able to use his lips and be able to swallow without gulping air. Tilt the beaker to the point where the liquid touches the upper lip leaving the child to do the rest, *do*

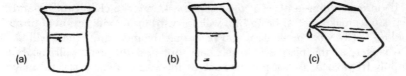

Figure 86
(a) A plastic beaker with a projecting rim is useful to start proper drinking.
(b) The beaker can be cut out on one side for the child's nose.
(c) Tilt the beaker this way for drinking.

not remove the beaker after each swallow, let it rest between the lips as otherwise the strong stimulus, which may result, can lead to you losing head and jaw-control. To start with, slightly thickened liquids such as yoghurt will be found easier, acid liquids are the most difficult owing to their tendency to increase the flow of saliva.

Never give the child who has drinking difficulties a cup or a beaker which has a spout as this will only make him relapse to primitive and abnormal sucking.

Drinking with a Polyester Tube

If we observe the progress of a *normal* child towards the ability to feed, it will be seen that sucking through a straw or tube is difficult and only comes at a late stage in his development; with cerebral palsied children it should not be attempted until fairly well co-ordinated drinking ability has been reached and then only to improve lip mobility or to help the athetoid or ataxic child who has difficulties in lifting the cup.

Use a thick walled polythene or polyester tube and one with a small inner diameter so that one suck allows a limited amount of liquid to come through and no air is gulped. The same method as that used in drinking from a cup should be used, the tube should be held and sucked by the lips alone, the jaws remaining closed with jaw-control if it is needed. To keep the tube in place and to avoid spilling, a beaker with a lid and a spout, similar to those used for patients in hospital, *in which the tube can be inserted* can be used. This will enable the child to put both his hands on the table round the beaker and help to stabilize him while he is sucking in the liquid through the tube.

THE FIRST STEPS TOWARDS SELF-FEEDING

The Normal Child.

Babies of a few weeks often rest a hand on their bottle while they are being fed, at about five to six months they hold the bottle with both hands, gradually the hands are brought in front of the child's face and he begins to look at them.

122

At about one month he starts to put one hand to his mouth, without being conscious that he is doing so, this is then followed by both hands and he starts to suck them.

At about six months when he starts to reach out and grasp, he will take a rusk to his mouth and suck it, but he will quickly drop it.

At about nine months he will take a rusk to his mouth but now in a deliberate way and will drop it only when he has had enough or his attention is distracted.

Some children at about eight to nine months begin to understand that the spoon and the food go together and will guide their mother's hand when she is feeding them with a spoon, others at this stage will help to guide a cup to their mouth. Babies, of course, differ considerably and some will never bother to help or will do so only when they are hungry.

Between the age of nine and twelve months a child will go through the stage of putting his hands into his food for the joy of squeezing it and will then smear it over his face and anything else that happens to be near. At this time the child will often snatch at the spoon when he is being fed but will only use it to bang on the table or to plunge it into the food; he is still unable to use a spoon to feed himself.

At about fifteen months he has the ability to grasp the spoon with his whole hand and to feed himself, for short periods however, and in a clumsy way. Finding difficulty in getting the food onto the spoon he will use his other hand to push the food on, dropping a great deal and turning the spoon over in his mouth in his effort to get the food off.

From now on through constant practise his abilities commence to improve fairly rapidly and by the time he reaches the age of two he has become proficient and most of the time usually insists on feeding himself.

The Cerebral Palsied Child

The athetoid child and the severely spastic quadruplegic child are often unable to reach the stage of being able to bring their hands before their face, much less to hold and to bring an object to their mouth; it must be appreciated that there is a clear difference between the problems of these two types of handicapped children. The athetoid child holds his arms away from his body, his head control and ability to focus his eyes are poor and his grasp is weak and ineffectual. The spastic quadruplegic child, whose whole body is involved, has both arms pressed against his side or over his chest with his hands clenched, usually with the thumbs tucked against the palms and has great difficulty in opening his fingers.

On the other hand the spastic diplegic child, – whose head, arms and hands are slightly affected, – at the age of about five months has little difficulty in reaching the stage of being able to take things to his mouth while lying on his back or on his tummy whilst he is at play. His difficulties, however, will be seen when he is sitting, as having no sitting balance he has to rely on his arms and hands for support and if he lifts up an arm to take his hand to his mouth or leans his head slightly backwards he is in danger of falling backwards.

123

The hemiplegic child will also be able, without much difficulty, to follow the normal developmental sequences leading to self-feeding. He however, will only use and look at his good hand and if his sitting position is poor, there will be an increase of 'associated reactions' in his affected arm and hand and he will experience difficulty when he starts to try to use a knife and a fork.

There is little point in forcing this child to use his affected hand unless he has a good grasp and can move his arm freely; the problem is that when trying to use a knife and fork the effort of cutting with the good hand, makes the affected arm and hand too stiff to handle the fork and to bring it to his mouth.

This is another example of an 'associated reaction' and it is one that can be overcome by allowing the child to eat in the manner adopted by some adults that is to say, first cutting up the food, then laying down the knife and using the same hand to lift the fork to the mouth; the child, however, should gradually learn to hold a fork in the affected hand and to apply pressure with his index finger. This is an isolated movement and he will have to learn to point with his index finger, keeping his other fingers bent before he can be taught to press down with a straight index finger.

We must not forget that even a *normal* child is not proficient in using a knife until he is about five years of age.

When the child is learning to feed himself, do not expect every mouthful to be a success and be prepared for a mess. A P.V.C. overall with long sleeves and a deep pocket at the bottom, and, one that fastens down the back is a 'must' at this time. Give him plenty of time and do not stint praise for achievement, otherwise he will soon lose interest and be happy to let you continue to feed him.

Until the child has acquired adequate sitting balance he must be controlled in his chair so that he has both hands free; the first essential of course is a suitable chair, when necessary use groin straps or a simple belt around the middle. In the case of the athetoid or ataxic child, a strap over the feet provides adequate stability and keeps the feet down, but adopt this method only as a temporary measure.

Start to prepare the child for self-feeding while he is still a young infant by bringing his arms forward to the bottle, refer again to figs. 78 (a)(b). In play encourage him to bring his hands to his mouth, i.e. mouthing, but *never* encourage thumb-sucking and later when you feed him with a spoon and a cup, try occasionally to open up his hands and put them on yours or around his beaker.

When your child has reached the stage where he wants to feed himself, analyse his difficulties carefully so that you will know exactly where he needs your help, do not bother him unduly, keep whatever help you feel you must give him to a minimum as this will lead to the maximum of effect, study figs. 87 to 93 and select whichever is most suitable.

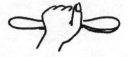
(a)

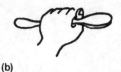
(b)

Figure 87
(a) *Wrong*. This grasp must be corrected as it will bring the spoon to the mouth in a wrong position, so that the food will have to be sucked off, instead of taken off with the lips.
(b) *Right*. The spoon needs to be held with a hand-grasp with the thumb going under the handle.

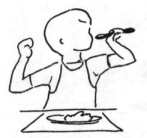
(a)

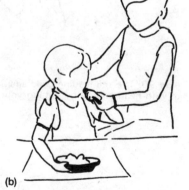
(b)

(c)

Figure 88
(a) *Wrong*. Self-feeding without control in hyperextension and in an asymmetrical pattern.
(b) *Right*. Self-feeding at the table, with control at the shoulder and supination of the hand holding the spoon.
(c) Adding supination to the hand by turning it out lightly from the root of the thumb.

125

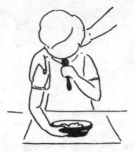

Figure 89. Right. A self-feeding child needs very little shoulder control. The hand, which he does not use, is put around the plate or bowl to keep it in front and to avoid extensor pattern.

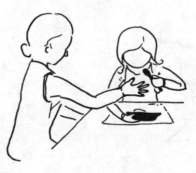

Figure 90. The self-feeding child sits across the corner of the table. You can help him with head control by putting your hand flat on his chest with pressure.

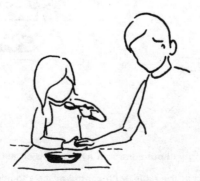

Figure 91. You can help your self-feeding child to avoid asymmetrical patterns by flexing his arm across his tummy on top or under the table, supinating his hand.

126

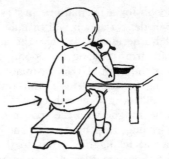

Figure 92. When trunk and head control are still difficult for the self-feeding child, sitting on a bench in riding fashion may be a good solution; if he tends to sit with a rounded back, he will need support at the lower part of his back.

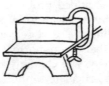

Figure 93. For support on lower back attach a block to the bench.

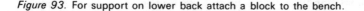

'Gadgets' for use in feeding must be kept to an absolute minimum; some of the following may however, prove to be of some use. For the child who has difficulty in getting the food onto a spoon, the steep side of a small bowl will be found more useful than a plate and by placing a non-slip mat underneath, it will be prevented from slipping; if a deep-sided plate can be managed, use the type that can have hot water put into the base to keep the food warm, as so many cerebral palsied children are slow eaters.

It should be remembered that an important part of self-feeding is to pick up your own knife, spoon and fork, cup or glass, no easy task for a cerebral palsied child; non-slip mats can now be bought in large sizes and will give additional help. When a child reaches the stage of learning left, right, top and bottom, reinforce this by getting him to place his own knife, fork and spoon in the correct position. Encourage him later to lay the places for the rest of the family including putting the glasses in the correct position.

Spoons, forks and knives can be fitted with plastic handles; these can be obtained in many 'do-it-yourself shops' and are available in three sizes and they can be bent according to your needs, see figs. 83(c)(d). 'Rubazote' tubing also makes a good temporary handle; do not forget to exchange the fitted spoon for a normal one just as soon as the child can hold it, in most cases a dessert spoon will usually be best.

Sometimes it will be necessary to help the self-feeding child with supination to keep him from placing the spoon in his mouth sideways instead of straight from the front. To do this place your hand lightly over the child's hand, turning the root of his thumb outwards with your own thumb, refer again to 88(b)(c); if he still cannot manage you may have to apply pressure on his tongue with the spoon.

When the child is feeding, help him with your hand to feed normally and most certainly avoid telling him what to do and do not be continually correcting him. For example, an open mouth, or a tongue thrust are part of a pattern of total extension, refer again to figs 84(a)(b). A jaw and tongue that deviate to one side are part of a general pattern of asymmetry, lack of head control means that the child does not have the stability necessary for the jaw, lips and tongue to work in a co-ordinated manner. If your child has the added problem of a high palate be very careful not to give him mushy or sticky foods such as bananas etc.

The early patterns of feeding are so closely linked to the development of future patterns of speech that any abnormal feeding patterns that are allowed to develop, or to persist will certainly affect the child's attempts to babble and later to make articulate sounds. By working closely with your speech therapist in attempting to prevent faulty feeding patterns, you will also be helping the child to develop the movements of the mouth, tongue and lips which he will need when he starts to speak.

Despite the difficulties, mealtimes should be enjoyable times for the child and for his parents – try not to become over-anxious as if you are he too will become over-anxious.

Remember that teaching your child to wash his hands before and after meals and to wipe his mouth and hands afterwards are important items in his programme of self-feeding.

DENTAL CARE

Children with cerebral palsy are usually very difficult to treat dentally; feeding problems especially those of chewing, make their teeth extremely susceptible to caries and the gums tend to become inflamed and swollen, dental care therefore is all the more important. Teeth cleaning also presents a problem due to their hypersensitive mouth and gums.

Advice on Cleaning Teeth

Before the milk teeth appear, or for the child who has not had previous treatment for a hypersensitive mouth, a good way of cleaning the gums is to use cotton wool dabbed in bicarbonate-of-soda or saline or even water. When the first teeth are coming through use a small infant-size toothbrush with water, gradually introducing toothpaste; remember that it is the mechanical brushing which keeps the child's mouth clean and healthy rather than the toothpaste.

When cleaning your child's teeth have him in a sitting position that enables him to have good head control.

With the small baby you will find it easier if you sit on a stool in front of the washbasin, with the baby on your lap or astride your knee. For the older child who can clean his own teeth, a stool close to the washbasin will enable him to rest his arms, giving him added stability.

If your child has difficulties in closing his mouth or is hypersensitive, jaw-control as used in feeding may be found helpful, refer again to fig. 82(a)(b). Remember that brushing the gums is just as important as brushing the teeth; always massage the gums towards the roots of the teeth. When you brush the outside of his gums and teeth use a circular movement, keeping his jaws closed, the head slightly flexed.

In time your child will learn to spit out the accumulated water, saliva and toothpaste. As a first step in learning to do this – that is before you open his jaw half-way to brush the inside of his gums and teeth – allow the accumulated water and so forth just to dribble out. It is important that you take care when doing this to see that your child's head does not push back, otherwise choking and gagging will occur.

The Electric Toothbrush

For children with cerebral palsy an electric toothbrush has considerable advantages. Independent studies in the United States and in Switzerland have shown that children with cerebral palsy who use electric toothbrushes have much healthier mouths than those who use ordinary brushes. There are two main reasons for this. Firstly, it is sometimes difficult for these children to make the correct brushing action with an ordinary toothbrush, whereas an electric toothbrush needing less manipulation, is usually easier to use. Secondly, these children can never brush as intensively and precisely by hand, whereas the electric toothbrush automatically massages thoroughly the gums and supporting tissue of the teeth; the tissues of the teeth of many of these children are notoriously spongy and swollen due to lack of the massage, which takes place whilst chewing solid foods.

Special Instructions on Dental Care

As dental surgery is difficult for the cerebral palsied child and for his dentist, it is very important that parents should be careful about the following points:

Cleaning the child's teeth after every meal.

Never giving the child snacks between meals.

Avoiding sugary foods, sweets and confectionery and soft drinks containing sugar; if the child does have sticky foods they should be restricted to mealtimes only and the teeth should be cleaned immediately afterwards. The child should be encouraged to eat detergent foods, for example, apples and carrots and so on, in preference to sugary foods.

It is important that the smallest toothbrush available be used as this enables you to brush the child's gums. Dentists stress that brushing the gums is even more important than brushing the teeth, as the gums are the supporting structure of the teeth and it is essential that the gums remain healthy. Food particles do collect around the edge of the gums with the result that bacteria multiply rapidly and the teeth start to decay, use dental floss to prevent food collecting between the teeth.

How often and from what age should the child have his teeth seen by his dentist? The answer is that the child is never too young, preferably he should be seen at the same time as other members of his family. If he attends at a sufficiently early age not only will he become accustomed to going to the dental surgery and will gradually become free from the fear which usually accompanies such visits, but the chances are that no treatment will be necessary for the first few visits, but these visits will be extremely useful in gaining the child's confidence. Finally every child should be seen by his dentist at least at six-monthly intervals.

Chapter 10

SPEECH

by Helen Mueller

SOME MAJOR STAGES IN SPEECH DEVELOPMENT OF THE *NORMAL* CHILD

The newborn expresses his needs through body-movements, facial expression and crying. These first sounds are totally nasal and monotonous at the beginning. Soon incidental sounds can be heard when the baby is moving, e.g. kicking, feeding or even falling asleep; he can hear the vowels and intonation of our speech, although in a very limited way.

During the third month when making "happy" sounds, his voice becomes less nasal and is produced more through his mouth, whilst crying or whining will remain nasal. Throaty sounds begin while the baby is lying mainly on his back.

At about four months the baby will start repetitive babbling, especially when he is left alone, this means that the sounds he is making are no longer purely accidental; it will be noticed that lip sounds occur more frequently when he turns onto his tummy. He will now start to turn to the source of the noise or sound and try to watch the mouth of the adult who is speaking.

At about six months when the baby progresses to sitting and begins to chew, (see chapter 9 on 'Feeding') lip and tongue sounds start to develop and rhythmical repetitions are more frequent and in this way chains of syllables are formed. Hearing is more differentiated and includes high frequencies, for example consonants.

At about eight months these syllable chains start to become more organised, i.e. broken up into single and double syllables such as ba-ba and reversed – a-ba. The variations in pitch and volume increase and a lot of self-imitation can be heard. In effect, the first little dialogue takes place.

From nine months onwards the first meaningful words are being used, even double syllabled words such as 'Mama', and imitation of rhythmical sounds combined with movement starts.

At about one year old the baby begins to understand such constantly used expressions as 'give it to Mummy', particularly if the sounds are

131

accompanied by gestures; he will begin to imitate adult speech by its intonation and thus starts his baby language.

Approaching the end of the second year, he will start to drop this baby language and will try to express himself by combining two words and eventually three-word phrases, but we must remember that at this time his understanding of language is far greater than his ability to express himself verbally. This accounts for the stuttering so often experienced between the age of two and three and which will be overcome with increasing use of the speech apparatus; it is most important that parents should recognise this and carefully avoid paying any real attention to it as it is merely an interim stage in progress towards speech.

At three years of age the child begins to start putting together simple sentences and is able to dissociate speech from gestures although to a limited extent, facial expressions and physical gestures generally accompany speech.

When we consider these developmental stages certain conclusions can be reached

- that speech develops out of movement and human contact.
- that body movements and sound production are linked in early infancy – later of course the child has sufficient control to hide his feelings and keep a straight face when speaking.
- that the foundations of speech are laid in infancy.
- that speech development does not start when the child says his first words but is dependent upon contact and the stimulations arising from his surroundings from birth onwards.

These facts must guide us when we are dealing with the speech problems of the cerebral palsied child.

When a child has a motor handicap his tools of speech, breathing, voice and articulation, facial expression and gestures will also frequently be involved.

SPEECH AND THE CEREBRAL PALSIED CHILD

When a parent speaks to a child who is spastic or ataxic the child will be slow in making any sound or assuming any facial expression; the athetoid child however will have almost an excess of facial expressions – grimacing and often an extreme of pitch and loudness in his voice. Each of these reactions is unusual and therefore strange to us and we are inclined to interpret them as indicating a lack of understanding or of intelligence; very likely we then give up trying to communicate with him or confine our talking to a minimum, probably thinking 'he does not seem to understand anyway'. By our reactions we are depriving the child of some of the most important stimulations and without which he cannot develop his language ability, involving thought patterns, speech and language.

If on the other hand the child shows no signs of any reaction to sounds and noises and you begin to be doubtful about his hearing ability, do not hesitate to take him to your doctor. In those rare cases where there is the possibility of hearing defect, early detection and training are of the utmost importance for language and speech development.

Preparation for Speech

If you handle your child as advised in the preceding chapters you will be helping him to improve his head and trunk control and at the same time helping him towards better feeding, thus giving him largely what he needs for the development of speech, i.e. an almost normal breathing pattern, co-ordination of the movements of his mouth and tongue and the possibility of making sounds without extra effort, leading to reasonably effortless articulation.

As in most other activities, the cerebral palsied child should be in a stable position and one which will not allow any grossly abnormal pattern to occur, fig. 94 shows a suitable position for a young child. Since we all make use of other senses in communication, such as lip-reading when we are listening to someone, your position when you are talking to the child is most important, for example, handling him in such a way that he has good head control. Always try to be in front of him at his eye-level, or slightly lower, so that he does not have to look up to you as this will probably throw him into a pattern of hyperextension; breathing and the effort to speak tend to cause this movement anyway, so guard against it by sitting or squatting down at the child's level, fig. 95 (b). You can also help your child before he gets ready to make sounds by controlling him from a suitable 'key-point', (see chapter 'Basic Principles of Handling') thus facilitating babbling or speech.

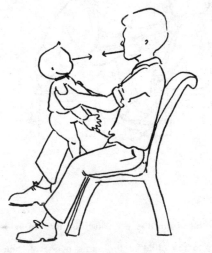

Figure 94. Speaking to the child so that he can watch your mouth without having to look up, control him from his upper arms or shoulders for a good head position.

133

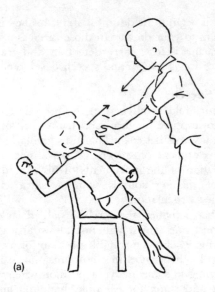

(a)

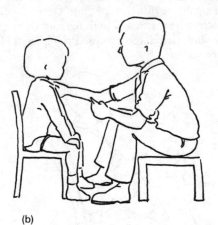

(b)

Figure 95
(a) Speaking to the child from above throws him into an extensor pattern making phonation difficult.
(b) *Right.* Speaking to the child at the same eye-level, helping him with head control from his shoulder or upper arm or by pressure on his lower chest with your flat hand.

For speech and babbling the baby needs to have delicate, co-ordinated movements of his lips, mouth and tongue; if these continue to function abnormally jaw control, see figs. 82 (a) (b) page 117 might be found helpful – with a baby this might consist of lip and tongue play to induce babbling in positions, such as those shown in figs. 78 (a) 79 (a) (b) in the chapter on 'Feeding'. Demonstrate with your own mouth and voice while you stroke lightly his upper or lower lip or move his tongue sideways or, with light control of his jaws, open and close his mouth to obtain chains of sounds such as 'ababa, bababa' etc. Never try to practise single sounds or certain mouth positions, as that would be unnatural and would tend to increase the child's tendency to block and get 'stuck'; these little babbling plays should be pleasant and short; at the same time we must remember that whilst results should be expected, we must not expect the child to succeed on the first occasion in imitating perfectly the sounds that you are making.

Some Common Problems

When your child reaches the age when specific sounds need to be made or, having been made, need to be corrected, do not tell or show him what or how to do it, nor expect him to learn from trying in front of a mirror, as his brain damage prevents him from translating auditory or visual commands (especially when they are 'mirror-like') into the correct movements.

It is important to remember that we should never practise isolated sounds with a cerebral palsied child. We must not forget that it is not lack of intelligence or effort which prevents the child from speaking correctly and that his difficulties are due to his *sensory-motor involvement;* undue persistence in our efforts will only increase the child's frustration by reinforcing his already frequent experiences of failure; you are performing a much more useful service by helping him to facilitate the necessary movements. This is admittedly a difficult undertaking when we consider the precision, fluency and speed of the movements necessary to produce articulate speech. In some cases of course it may be essential to seek the assistance of a speech therapist.

Speech problems caused by abnormal breathing cannot be corrected through 'blowing' exercises as these would only increase spasticity and in such cases it is advisable to consult your physiotherapist or your speech therapist.

If the child's voice is weak it is not a good idea to tell him to speak louder as he can only do so with great effort and this will merely mean an increase in spasticity. Aim rather for better trunk and head control as this may help his breathing and in turn should improve the volume of his voice. An open mouth is always a passive mouth, whether it is due to hyperextension or lack of muscle tone, and you will need the help of your physiotherapist or speech therapist to deal with this problem. You can practise mouth closure at home, during meal times and sleeping times while watching for good head control, pressure above the upper lip, (see the chapter on 'Feeding') can be applied in between times, or you can stroke his lower lip two or three times; there is no need to say anything when you are doing this. Remember that mouth closure is essential for breathing through the nose, breathing whilst swallowing, articulation, dental health and dental occlusion.

Mouth closing will not improve by continually telling the child to keep his mouth closed and must be treated as part of his overall disability, thumb-sucking will certainly counteract your efforts and, if it is essential, should be replaced by a 'dummy' as this, of course, can be discarded so much more easily in the very early stages of its use. A helpful method is to try to direct the child's interest towards a toy, or some absorbing activity which might be going on around him. Mouthing – (experimenting with hands and objects at and in the mouth) is an entirely different thing and most certainly has its place in the development of speech; it represents an important sensory-motor experience and should be encouraged in the young handicapped baby, see chapter on "Feeding".

Remember that all these preparations for speaking must be integrated into the daily life of a child in early infancy, in the hopes that when he is ready to talk, what we have described as his 'speech tools' will be available and under reasonable control.

Sensory Input
It has already been pointed out that the baby receives and takes in speech, including facial expressions and gestures with all his senses, not merely that of hearing. Because of his motor problems your baby may be deprived of part of these sensory experiences, therefore you will have to try to bring them to him; do not, however, bombard him with sensory stimuli as a young child's perception is not yet organised, i.e. is not yet able to distinguish the important from the unimportant, or to put things into proper sequence; the brain damaged child might be slow in maturation of perception anyway, and if, in your natural anxiety, the rate of progress you wish him to make is too fast, he will merely become frustrated, retire into himself, or lose interest altogether.

A baby learns and forms concepts by mouthing, handling, manipulating, playing and listening to your talking about the objects you are showing him. Use the parts of his body, simple elementary toys, the things that you use when feeding, bathing, dressing him and so on. Do not expect the young child to maintain his interest and to want to take part in such play for more than a short time, nor expect any immediate verbal reaction from him, let alone imitation of your talking – stop while he still has fun and he will be eager to go on the next time.

It is *normal* for a young child just to listen, watch, manipulate and even laugh but not 'say' anything until possibly many days later. As play is the form in which he will absorb and learn during the first few years of his

136

life, make the occasion one of play rather than a teaching situation, use objects of different colours, shapes, textures and sounds, even tastes and temperatures; name each of them and talk a little about them and what they are used for; *all this will help to develop the sensory avenues which are necessary for the formation of language.* From the development of the *normal* child we have learned that rhythm plays an important part in the early stages of development, therefore for the cerebral palsied child reinforce rhythmical verbal play with rhythmical body movements, e.g. clapping hands; an essential activity if the child is to learn to use his hands one independently of the other. Later on of course nursery rhymes with suitable actions and words should be introduced.

Attempting Speech

When the child attempts babbling or speech but without very much success, all the joy will be taken out of it for him if you try immediately to correct his attempts; *remember that it takes the normal child about five years to reach a reasonable level of speech.* The pleasure of playing with speech is a very important factor in speech development and must be taken into account. Let the child play with speech, let him experiment before trying to help him, be careful, however, not to become too excited at his first successful attempts and not to start urging him to repeat; too much fuss makes a child withdraw just as easily as neglect or constant correction.

Look upon his efforts to speak as being normal and let him see by experience that speech in day-to-day living is necessary and of course interesting.

Gestures

During the first year of life gestures are essential. When you go about your daily activities speak to your child mainly about those activities that directly concern him; name objects first, then the verbs for the activities and so on and eventually construct little sentences. We must not, however, run the risk of over-emphasizing the importance of gestures as otherwise the child might not develop beyond them either on the receptive or the expressive side; the danger would then be that he would never learn to dissociate language from gesture.

We must give the handicapped child plenty of opportunity to express himself, no matter how fragmentary or unsuccessful his first attempts may prove to be. If we keep reading every need or wish from the expression in his eyes or from his gestures; if we answer every question for him; if we always speak for him, he will have no need nor incentive whatsoever to talk and the valuable and sensitive phase for the development of speech will pass unused. Ask him simple questions, letting him feel by your intonation and facial expressions that you expect a reply and one that lies within his mental and verbal capacity. Ignore his gesturing or nodding of the head more and more and, this is most important, do not forget to be patient in waiting for his answers, as they will often be slow and delayed in coming.

Personal Interaction

We hope that what we have said will leave you in no doubt as to the importance of close contact between yourself and your child, as you help him to build up *'inner language'* which is so essential for his future speech development. Television, radio, records, tapes and so on however excellent their presentation, have only a very limited value and place in the child's speech development and can never replace personal contact as you help your child build up his vocabulary; while, for example, reading a book do so by speaking slowly, explaining any new words, stopping frequently to repeat and explain their meaning – personal touches that are so important but impossible when technical devices are used.

In our efforts to help the child to form concepts we should start by teaching him about his own body, the objects around him in his cot, his playpen and so on. By these means gradually widening his horizon by talking about familiar objects he knows and uses in his room. Later take him to the window and talk about the familiar scene outside, let him see the postman coming in to deliver the letters, the milkman with the milk and so forth. He should then be ready to look at the first simple picture books representing objects with which he is familiar, from these he can go on to pictures that represent everyday simple situations.

When choosing books be sure to take the child's limited experience into account. A child who is fairly immobile or has, for example, never been to the country cannot be expected to recognise the farm animals in the pictures he is shown.

Choose books carefully, finding ways and means to enlarge the child's world despite his physical handicap. When you show him things in the picture books, name them, talk about their use, their special characteristics, their colours and so on, gradually introducing nouns, adjectives and verbs, remember, however, that this cannot be done all at once; later, as he progresses, a children's picture dictionary may be found useful. Have short pleasant sessions and you will find that the child himself will keep asking to look at the pictures over and over again; 'feed' him a little at one time so that he can absorb and stay interested.

The age at which articulation of a specific consonant, or the use of the first word emerges, must never be of primary concern to us as it is known that it differs greatly among children. Remember that what will really count in the future of the cerebral palsied child is not merely perfect articulation, but the ability to use language and thus be able to speak without undue physical effort and tenseness and in this way being easily and clearly understood.

I have tried in this chapter to stress the importance of *early sensory motor preparation* and the part the parent can play in helping the child towards effective speech.

Chapter 11

CARRYING

How does a *normal* five month old baby react when we bend forward to pick him up? He immediately anticipates our intention by lifting his head and reaching out towards us with his arms, often kicking his legs in excitement. Carrying him presents no problems as he automatically holds on or puts his arms around our neck, his legs open easily and while we shift his position, to make holding easier for ourselves, he adjusts himself to our handling. If he should lose his balance, he will immediately grasp hold of us to save himself. When we put him down we can see that he keeps his head, shoulders and arms forward until the *last* moment.

The cerebral palsied child cannot automatically reach out towards us as we bend forward to pick him up as he is pulled away by his abnormal patterns of posture and movement. The excitement of being picked up, or even his own effort to participate in the movement, results in the child becoming stiff, his head and shoulders are pulled backwards or forwards, both these movements reinforce the tight bending of his arms, often with fisted hands, sometimes his head is also turned to one side with an effect on his whole body. When we put him down we can see that his head, shoulders and arms, in that order, are the *first* parts of him to touch the support if he is not properly controlled.

It is therefore obvious that, if we are to avoid difficulties when we carry the cerebral palsied child, we must first assess his problems, not only to find out how much help he needs, but also to see how much of the movement he is capable of doing himself, controlling him adequately but only where necessary *before* lifting him and using the *same control* to put him down.

Far too many cerebral palsied children, long after they are babies, are carried as shown in fig. 96. Not only is this bad for the child emotionally, it does not give him a chance, if supported in this way, to do anything for himself. It also robs him of the opportunity to see what is going on around him.

Let us first consider the lifting and carrying of the young spastic child who is predominantly *extended*.

The first and most important point to remember is to sit the child up symmetrically *before* lifting him, bending him well forward at the hips, as shown in figs. 97 (a) to (d), giving the child a good base for being carried; the drawing also illustrates how your support can gradually be

139

reduced. Held in this way it will be seen, firstly, that the child, if he has the ability to grasp, is able to put his arms around his mother's neck and, secondly, he is able to make use of what ability he has to balance, he also has an opportunity to look around – fig. 98 shows a simple way of carrying the young spastic child around the house.

Let us now consider the lifting and carrying of the young spastic child who is predominantly *flexed*, and who in all positions has his head pulled onto his chest, arms bent, spine rounded, often finding it difficult to extend his hips, the 'position' in which he is carried may reinforce his difficulties; when he is at home try holding him as illustrated in figs. 99 (a) (b). This will help him extend his hips, stimulating him to extend his head and body – be careful to see if the child has rather stiff legs, that you can keep them apart *and* turned out.

Fig. 100 (a) illustrates how a *normal* child who has sitting balance, i.e. head and trunk control, is carried, it will be seen that the outside leg is bent. In the cerebral palsied child, one leg is always more apt to bend than the other, especially if, as we have already described, the head is turned predominantly to one side, i.e. where the right leg is more apt to bend he should be held on the left side of his mother. In practice, this is not always possible as most of us are predominanently right-handed or left-handed, fig. 100 (b) shows how this difficulty can be overcome.

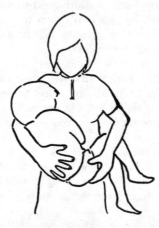

Figure 96. A cerebral palsied child carried as a baby, completely supported and unable to look around. Note when carrying the child in this way the tendency is to pull him towards you, especially at the hips. This is an abnormal position and similar to that which the child adopts when lying on his back.

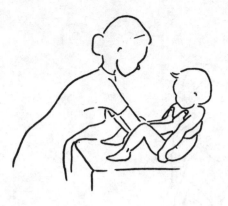
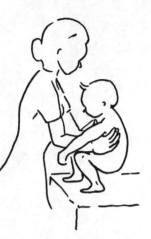

(a) and (b)

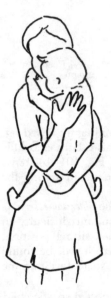
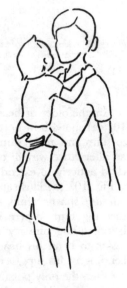

(c) and (d)

Figure 97
One of the ways of lifting a young *spastic child* who is predominantly *extended*.
(a) and (b) First bring him up into a sitting position, controlling him at the shoulders, holding him under the top of his arms which should be lifted and turned out. This will help to bring his head and arms forward and facilitate the bending of his hips and knees, your forearms helping to keep his knees apart.
(c) and (d) Having taken the child into the sitting position lift him and hold as illustrated. First place his arms over your shoulders and then part his legs to put around your waist. As the child learns to balance gradually reduce your support.

141

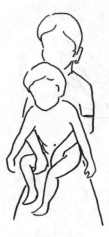

Figure 98. A simple way of carrying a young *spastic* child around the house. Description of control is described under 'swinging the child in the air'. (Fig. 19 (a), chapter 3)

For the older or heavier spastic child who is predominantly flexed fig. 101 (a) shows how both parents can hold the child, this is both enjoyable for him and at the same time is a form of treatment. Fig. 101 (b) shows an alternative way of control by one parent which results in getting the child actively to extend.

Fig. 102 (a) illustrates the *incorrect* way of *lifting* the *older more severely extended* spastic child and figs. 102 (b) (c) the resultant difficulty in carrying him. Where it is difficult to get him into a sitting position, before lifting him try rolling him onto his side where it will be found easier to bend his head and shoulders forward and so to facilitate the bending of his hips, see fig. 103.

Often the only possible way to carry the severely affected spastic child of this type, who is rather heavy, is over your shoulder, fig. 104 (a) shows the *incorrect* way and fig. 104 (b) the *correct* way to do this.

Unlike the spastic child who is stiff, finding difficulty in moving or adjusting his position to being moved, the athetoid child has uncontrolled and continuous unwanted (involuntary) movements, he has the tendency when lying on his back to press his head, shoulders and arms against the support, hips often bent, legs bent and apart. Our handling when lifting and carrying him must be steady and firm, giving him as much stability as possible, see figs. 105 (a) – (d).

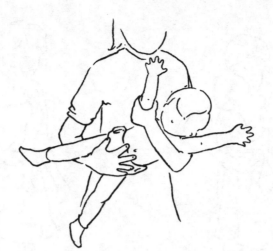

(a)

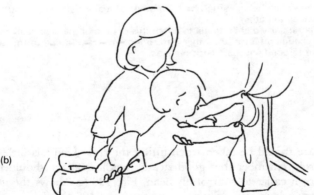

(b)

Figure 99
Carrying the *spastic child* who is predominantly *flexed*.
(a) If held extended on his side against you, you can straighten his back while at the same time stopping the pulling down and bending of his arms, and keeping his legs apart lessens his tendency to bend at the hips and cross his legs.
(b) An alternative and more active position, facilitating the lifting of the head, extension of the back, and the reaching out of both arms enabling the child, as you carry him, to explore his surroundings.

143

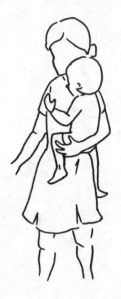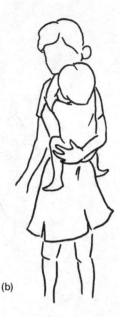

(a)   (b)

Figure 100
(a) The *normal* child being carried by his mother bends his left leg (the outside leg)
and straightens the other.
(b) If a cerebral palsied child tends to adopt this pattern of the legs in all positions,
instead of changing him to the other arm, bring him forward and in this way you
will be able to bend and part both his legs.

Extra care should be taken when lifting the child who has little or no
head control, remember that good steady handling at the shoulders and
arms makes it easier to control his head. Fig. 106 (a) shows the *incorrect*
way to carry a low toned 'floppy' child, and fig. 106 (b) the *correct* way.
There are now available a number of types of 'Kiddy Carriers' and
'Baby Slings', which are used by mothers when it is necessary for them
to have their hands free, for example, when out shopping. Some are
designed to be slung on the front or side, others over the back. Fig. 107
illustrates the type of 'Kiddy Carrier' that can be used with or without
a frame. If you are contemplating buying a 'Kiddy Carrier' or 'Baby
Sling', do be sure to try them out *before* buying. Your child must have
fairly good head control and the ability to adjust to sudden changes in
movement if he is to be able to sit in a 'Baby Sling', or he will slip down
into lying, and it will be impossible for you to control him.

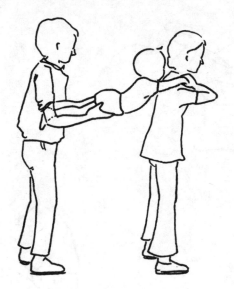

(a)

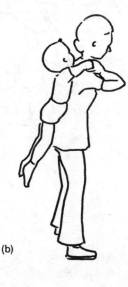
(b)

Figure 101
(a) The older heavier *spastic* child who is predominantly flexed, carried by both parents. The legs are held apart and out at the hips, the feet flat against your body. When the hips are really straight and the child has no spasm, push up with your thumbs from the bottom of the buttocks, stimulating the back and head to extend actively.
(b) Shows how one parent can hold the child to encourage extension.

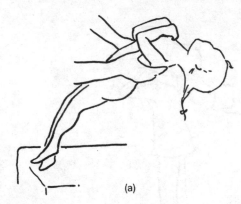

(a)

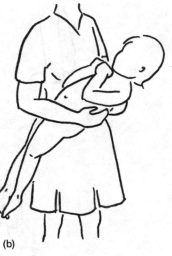

(b)

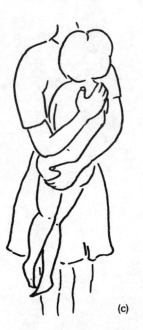

(c)

Figure 102
(a) *Incorrect way to lift* the older more severely *extended* child from the lying position.
(b) and (c) Illustrate the problems in carrying that result, i.e. difficulty in bending his hips, bending and opening his legs, and the impossibility of putting his arms over your shoulders.

146

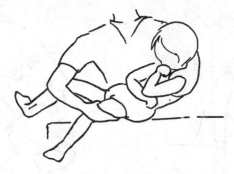

Figure 103. The *spastic* child with *strong extensor spasms* may be easier to lift if you roll him slightly to one side as this will make it easier to bring his head and shoulders forward and to bend his hips.

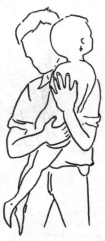

(a)

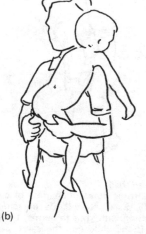

(b)

Figure 104
(a) *Incorrect way to carry* a heavy severely affected *spastic* child. Holding in this way, the arms are pulled together and this results in the legs becoming stiffer, closer together and often crossed. It is then difficult to bend the hips and part the legs.
(b) By keeping the arms over your shoulder and holding the legs high up on the thighs, it is possible to keep the legs apart and turn them out, and it will be much easier to carry the child.

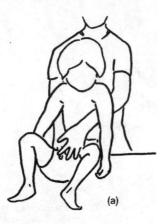
(a)

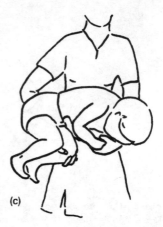
(c)

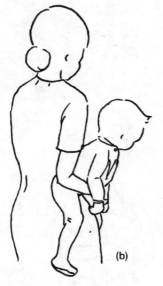
(b)

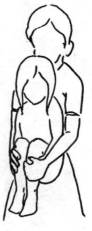
(d)

Figure 105
(a) Lift the *athetoid* child by placing your arms under his arms, your hands on his body, as illustrated. By pressing your hands gently in, and at the same time pushing with your forearms, his head and arms will come forward.
(b) If the child has the same pattern of head, trunk and arms as in (a) but in addition has very stiff extended hips and legs, control him in the same way as in fig. (a) and at the same time turn him on his side *before* you lift him and you will find it easier to bend his hips and part and bend his legs.
(c) A good way to carry a young *athetoid* child. He has both flexion and stability at his hips and by having him leaning slightly forward and placing a hand on his chest you are able to keep his arms forward. This will facilitate the extension of his head and back while at the same time his hips will remain bent.
(d) A simple way of carrying an *athetoid* or a *'floppy'* child around the house. Description of control described under 'swinging the child in the air' - (Fig. 19(b) Chapter 3)

148

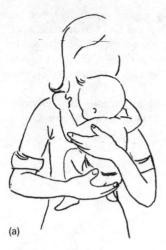

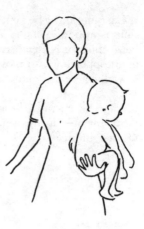

(a)

(b)

Figure 106
(a) The *incorrect* way to carry a *'floppy'* child who has no head or trunk control –
he is completely passive.
(b) The *correct* way to carry a *'floppy'* child his legs are bent and together and firm
support is given at the hips – this gives him sufficient stability to start actively to
extend his head and back.

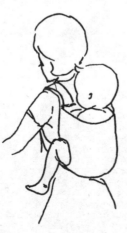

Figure 107. 'Kiddy Carrier' for carrying young child; illustrated without frame.

149

Carrying must be kept to a minimum, this applies especially when the child is at home; one is often tempted to carry the child as it saves time, but it must be remembered that each time we do so we are depriving him of an opportunity to move on his own. Even if a child is unable to crawl or walk there are many alternative ways of moving around, see chapter 14.

All children must be given the opportunity to explore their environment, for only in this way will they gain the experiences that are so vital to their future.

Chapter 12

PRAMS, PUSH-CHAIRS, AND CHAIRS

In this chapter we shall deal with some of the problems that may arise when the child is in a pram, push-chair or chair, attempting to give some practical advice on these problems, and pointing out the ways in which they can be dealt with.

As each child has his own problems and difficulties, and no two children are alike, there is no perfect solution, it is only by careful observation of each child that the correct choice of pram, push-chair or chair can be made. We shall use the fundamental principles of looking at the child as a whole, realising what movements he should be able to make, and therefore how he should sit and move when he is in his push-chair, and understanding the reasons for his difficulties.

It is essential that a child should at all times be given the opportunity to use whatever potential abilities he has, allowing him to control and adjust his position by himself whenever possible, and in this way learning to get his own balance. Therefore, the outside support given him and the adjustments advised should be restricted to the absolute minimum, just sufficient to prevent him from going wrong, without interfering with his own movements, and removing any outside support immediately it is no longer required.

PRAMS
When selecting a pram remember to take into account the child's difficulties, not only when he is sitting in the pram while it is stationary, but also while it is moving. Select a pram in which the child can sit well. The cerebral palsied child has a valuable opportunity giving him mental stimulation to see and hear when sitting out of doors in his pram. Nothing can be more conducive to the child's mental inertia than lying flat on his back, gazing at the hood of the pram, or at the sky.'

What are the difficulties that may face the child when he is sitting in his pram? He may lack head control, thus being unable to sit unless he is completely supported. He may push his head against the pillow whilst straightening his hips and legs, causing him to slip down, he may bend too far forward, allowing his whole trunk to fall forward, making it impossible for him to lift his head and to look around, or he may collapse and fall over to one side. To avoid any or all of these happening, it is important that the child is supported where necessary when sitting in the

151

pram, some of the foam shapes mentioned in the paragraph on chairs may be found useful for placing in the pram for extra support. Some children may have better support if a ply-wood sitting frame is made i.e. chair back and seat, the firm base giving them more support.

PUSH-CHAIRS

Many of the difficulties mentioned in connection with prams will also be met with when using a push-chair; there are, however, additional problems depending on the child's degree of spasticity or athetosis.

When looking for a push-chair for a spastic child we should ask ourselves such questions as – is the seat or the back of the chair too soft, making it impossible for the child to sit up and back at his hips, or making it impossible for him to lift his head owing to the rounding of his spine and the downward pressure from his shoulders? Is the foot-rest the correct height, not too high nor too low? If it is too high the child may push against it with his feet, his head and body go backwards and his legs straighten and tend to cross, with the result that he will slip forward. If, on the other hand it is too low, only his toes will come into contact with the support, this will have the effect of making him extend his legs and hips. Care should be taken to see that the seat and the foot-rest do not become lop-sided, due to uneven pressure of weight by the child who is inclined to take all his weight over to one side.

Let us now look at the questions that we should ask ourselves when looking for a push-chair for an athetoid child, bearing in mind that he often has total patterns of movement that either flex or extend his body, and in addition he may have strong intermittent spasms. Is the seat or the back of the chair too hard, causing too much stimulation and resulting in him pushing back with his head and shoulders and his hips and legs extending? Is the angle of the seat correct, or is the front, being much higher than the back, making his hips flex excessively? Is the seat too wide or are the sides too low, resulting in a tendency to increased asymmetry and poor balance?

Some of the following points may help when you are adapting the push-chair. Make sure, especially for many of the spastic children, that the *back-rest* is firm, we have used a thin piece of plywood with a layer of foam-rubber covered with washable material. Make sure that the seat is firm, here again a piece of thick foam-rubber is useful. For some children a thin cushion of small foam-chips without a cover prevents slipping. Some children push themselves backwards when their feet come in contact with a firm non-slip surface, in these cases it is advisable to dispense with a foot-rest until they have learned not to push back. If the child's feet turn in excessively, his hips and knees will also turn in, and most likely one leg will bend more than the other, fig. 125, page 171, shows how, by the use of two padded blocks screwed onto a chair, the legs can be kept apart and the hips turned out. The push-chair can be similarly adapted.

If groin straps are needed for the child who has no sitting balance, make sure that the angle of the straps across the groins is correct, the straps should be tied downwards and backwards. If they are too high, or tied too tightly, they can cause the child to have a spasm in the muscles of the hips, so that he falls forwards and cannot lift his head. Another possible and painful effect might be that the child will hollow his lower spine and at the same time throw his shoulders and arms back.

For the child who is afraid of falling forwards, the normal type of tray-fitment or a broad piece of webbing will give more confidence, the webbing need not be attached to the child, it can be stretched in front of his waist. Having the sides of the push-chair blocked-in adds to his feeling of security. The lack of stability, balance and head control of an athetoid child can be partially counteracted by placing a small sandbag by the side of his hips, or a wooden rail across the end of the arm-rests to hold onto.

The Baby Buggy

We have been recommending the 'Baby Buggy' see fig. 108, to parents of athetoid children who have strong intermittent spasms into extension. The sloping canvas back of this chair helps to inhibit this abnormal pattern by keeping the head and shoulders well forward. As soon as the child is able to modify this pattern the back rest should be made firmer by reinforcing it with an extra-wide piece of webbing. If later the seat becomes too deep and short, an inflatable cushion can be used. When the child is ready to sit in a more upright position, two inflatable cushions covered in a washable material, as illustrated fig. 109, will provide a firmer seat and back rest.

However satisfactory the 'Baby Buggy' may be, a few minor adjustments may have to be made. In some cases the foot-rest and band, to keep the feet down, will be too narrow, and the child may find it difficult to control the involuntary bending at his hips, or may be inclined to straighten his legs and press them together. Some of these problems can, to some extent, be dealt with by using wide bands of material with 'Velcro' sewn onto the ends and attached to the canvas of the chair with a strip of 'Velcro'.

Buggy Major

For the older child the 'Buggy Major' is a useful and light chair. If the child has very poor trunk control an extra insert can be bought which fits over the back of the chair with two flaps that come around the side of the body and the front, see fig. 110, when no longer needed this extra support can be removed.

A child may feel nervous in his push-chair, perhaps because his balance is poor and he is afraid of falling forwards, or because he has the type of push-chair in which he sits with his back to his mother, and to see her has to look up and back, again disturbing his balance. Given the choice

153

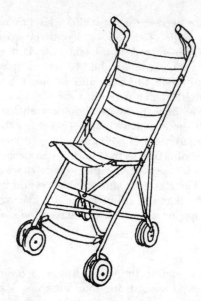

Figure 108. 'Baby Buggy'

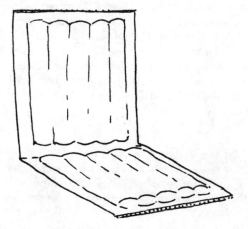

Figure 109. Terry-towelling cover sewn down the middle to form two pockets to take the two inflatable cushions.

between two otherwise suitable push-chairs (other than in cases where the 'Baby Buggy' is recommended) choose the one in which your child sits facing you and preferably one with a bar in front to hold onto.

Obviously there is no ideal push-chair, therefore before finally deciding try a number of different types. Choose a basically simple model, as this is always easier to adapt. When you are buying a push-chair do not merely choose one from a catalogue. First get professional advice from your therapist, and then take your child to the shop and try out the various models, rather than finding out the problems after you have bought the push-chair. Watch to see how your child balances not only when the push-chair is stationary, but also when it is being wheeled. Many shops will allow you to have a push-chair on approval – take advantage of this service.

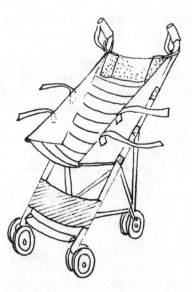

Figure 110. 'Buggy Major' showing adaptations – pillow with foam on each side of the head-piece – seat-insert with straps – band to prevent feet from slipping backwards.

CHAIRS

What are the basic requirements for a suitable chair? One that enables the child to achieve good head and trunk control so that he can balance, giving him every chance to move forwards at his hips and shoulders in order to bring his arms forward to use his hands. A suitable chair should be simple and one that can easily have the required adjustments made. We have found, when possible, that a *normal* child's armchair or, for the older child, a wooden kitchen chair, or a wooden box, not varnished or polished, is the best.

We strongly believe that no child should spend long periods in a chair. The severely handicapped child, if he is to sit at all, will have to be completely supported and often tied in; this is equivalent to us sitting, for example, in a small seat in a cinema for about three hours without getting up, although we are continually shifting our position, when we do get up we are very stiff indeed. It is obvious therefore that a child, who is completely tied in and unable to move as hours pass, will not only become very stiff, but will also be in danger of developing contractures or deformities. It is for this reason that such children should spend part of the day on the floor in a variety of positions, and be given the opportunity of moving around freely.

If the child is severely handicapped, the chair must not only be easily adaptable, but be of a sensible height, so that handling the child is made easier. A child with no trunk control must be adequately supported if he is to control his head; but for the child who is beginning to get sitting balance, it is important that he should sit on a stool or box without a back-rest, i.e. with no support, so that he can practise balancing and learn to regain his balance.

Think carefully of the occasions when the child will be using the chair. For example, for a very severely handicapped child who has reached the age of five, it is far better to have a small wooden armchair that can be adapted to his particular difficulties, so that he can join in the activities of his friends who will, most likely, be sitting around a small table or playing on the floor, small castors can easily be fixed to the back legs of the chair to make it mobile. The child may need a high-chair for meal-times but this should not be used at other times, unless it is the type of high-chair which doubles-up as a low-chair with a small table attachment. Whenever possible he should sit in the chairs, including the armchairs, that are in general use in his home; the corner of a sofa makes a safe seat for a severely handicapped small child who continually throws himself backwards when sitting.

There are many children who, using their hands for support, may sit well while reading or watching television, but have insufficient balance for activities requiring the use of both hands, e.g. for eating and dressing, and need more support during these activities. When such a child is beginning to dress or undress himself, a stool against the corner of the wall, or a low chair – with or without arms and large enough for him to move about on – is most satisfactory. Some children feel safer sitting on a bench-type stool as it provides a larger surface on which to support themselves, and it has the added advantage that, when dressing, they can have their clothes within easy reach. They feel safe with their feet on the ground, and when they have to stand up or sit down can do so without falling over.

For the child who cannot sit in a chair because he pushes back with his head, shoulders, arms and trunk, making it impossible to bend his hips, we have found that control from the head and shoulders is very helpful, see fig. 111 (a), this shows how by using a towel or broad piece of webbing we can control the pushing *forwards* of the head and shoulders, fig. 111 (b) shows how by using a towel or broad piece of webbing we can control the pushing *back* of the head and shoulders. If a child is constantly falling over to one side, he will need support in two directions to help him to sit straight; watch to see on which side he is taking his weight, and feel under which arm you get the most downward pressure. Figs. 112 (a) (b) illustrate these points and the means by which they can be overcome.

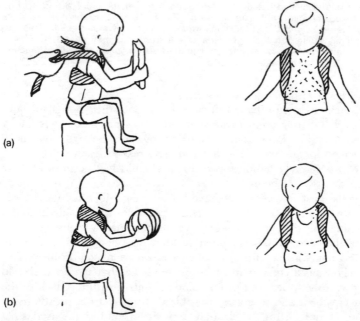

(a)

(b)

Figure 111
(a) Towelling or webbing controlling the *pushing forward of the head and shoulders.* Place the towel across the back, under the arms, over the shoulders and tie or fasten with 'Velcro'.
(b) Towelling or webbing controlling the *pushing back of the head and shoulders.* Place the towel around the back of the neck, over the shoulders, under the arms and tie or fasten with 'Velcro' behind the neck. Note: the dotted line in sketch is an extra band that can be added to stop the towel slipping.

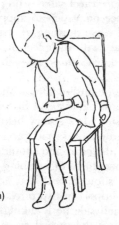
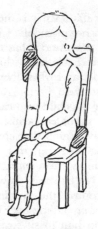

(a)   (b)

Figure 112
(a) The child sits asymmetrically, no weight is taken on the left buttock; the head, right shoulder and right side of the trunk bend and push down on that side.
(b) A sand bag is placed beside the left buttock to get the child sitting symmetrically. A piece of foam-rubber is placed behind and slightly to the outside of the right shoulder to keep the shoulder forward and slightly towards the left. This may not completely straighten the right side of the trunk but may go a long way to stopping it getting progressively worse. The foam rubber pads are kept in place by 'Velcro' attached to the pads and to the chair.

Most athetoid children have difficulty in keeping their heads still and this makes it hard for them to look at what they are doing, wearing a beret with lead-shot inserted into it will sometimes help to give more stability when, for instance, they are trying to read or write. The sitting balance of the severely handicapped athetoid child will be improved by the use of this type of beret.

During the past few years we have been giving thought to the basic shapes and materials in which a chair could be designed, and the covering materials that are available. We did this mainly to find suitable chairs for the severely handicapped child, with poor head and trunk control and therefore no sitting balance – always a major problem.

When choosing a chair it must be remembered that the child should be sitting with the lower part of his spine in contact with the back of the chair, his hips bent and whenever possible with his feet flat on the floor. Half-lying is not sitting, and such a position should be used as a temporary measure only and for as short a time as possible. Another consideration, when choosing a chair, is the need to bear in mind the present and future activities of the child when sitting in it. With the help of the sketches, figs. 113-136, let us consider some of the shapes and materials available, discussing their merits and suitability, or otherwise, for children with different handicaps.

The 'Bean-Bag' Chair

This chair is suitable for the severely handicapped child, it is filled with polystyrene pellets and foam chips and has an inner and outer covering of sail-cloth, the outer covering has a zip-fastener and can be removed for washing; sail-cloth being strong and durable is an excellent covering. We have tried various alternative materials, including those that can be washed down without being removed, but these materials have proved rather hot and sticky. The filling of the 'Bean Bag' enables you to mould it into any shape that you require, giving extra suppoort to the child where necessary, no extra straps or outside supports are needed, see fig. 113 (a). For severely handicapped children who find it difficult to bring their arms forward in a 'Bean-Bag' chair, placing them in side-lying, as a first step, may prove helpful, see fig. 113 (b).

These chairs are very comfortable, and if you sit in one you will appreciate how quickly you relax and how conducive they are to sleep, your child will also be quick to realise this. It is important to remember that the softness of this chair makes adjustment of the sitting position difficult for the child. For this reason use the chair only for short periods during the day, usually choosing times when your child wants to watch T.V., or read a book and so forth, see figs. 113 (c) (d).

'Bean-Bag' chairs are often used by mothers when treating or playing with a baby or a young child, or when giving oral therapy. The 'Bean-Bag' chair also serves the purpose of providing a comfortable chair for any member of the family when not being used by the child.

Please note that we do *not recommend* the use of this chair for the very inactive, floppy or flexed child. We repeat *only* use this chair for the severely extended handicapped child who is unable to learn any form of postural control and then *only* for short periods.

Inflatable Chairs

If you look around the shops you will see various inflatable chairs in such shapes as a triangle, a round seat for very small children, and a replica of an adult's armchair. We will not discuss the latter chair as we have not found it useful for the under fives.

Triangle Inflatable Chair

We have found this chair, see fig. 114 most useful for the athetoid child who has strong spasms that push him back when sitting, as the lack of stimulation on the buttocks, due to the hollow in the seat, minimises this strong pattern of extension, and the triangle shaped back helps to keep the head and shoulders forward. The deep front of the seat makes it easier to have the legs bent and together, counteracting the side abduction of the bent legs often found in athetoid children. A word of warning about inflatable chairs; as these chairs are generally rather light, for safety they should only be placed where there is additional stable support.

159

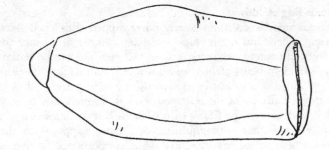

(a)

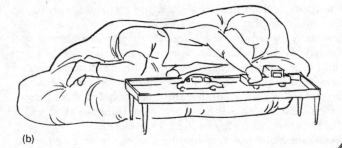

(b)

(c)

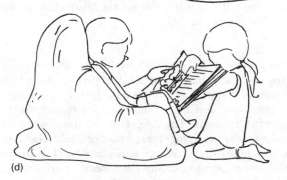

(d)

Figure 113. The Bean Bag Chair

160

Please note that we do *not recommend* this chair for the very flexed spastic or floppy child as it reinforces their abnormal pattern of total flexion.

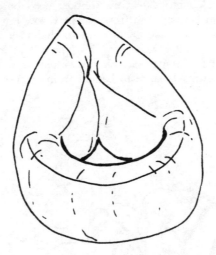

Figure 114. Inflatable Triangle Chair

Round Inflatable Chair

This chair is of use for small children *only*, it is small and light and can be placed in an armchair, or pram, but *not* of course, in a push-chair. Some parents have found this chair useful when feeding or playing with their child – see fig. 115.

Please note that we do *not recommend* that you leave a child unsupervised in this type of chair, as there is no means by which he can be given additional support.

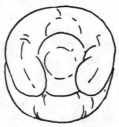

Figure 115. Round Inflatable Chair

'Safa' Bath Seat

This was originally designed by a father for use in the bath by his handicapped child, see chapter 7, fig. 62 (d). We have also found it useful as an ordinary seat for a young child who is just beginning to get sitting balance, and it is particularly useful for the young spastic hemiplegic child.

161

This type of seat gives the child a feeling of security as his feet are on the ground; it also has the advantage that there is when necessary a metal bar for him to hold onto. No extra support need be given, and when needed a table can be placed in front for play. We have found that the best way is to suspend the seat between two chairs see fig. 116.

Please note that we do *not recommend* this type of seat for any child with strong extensor or flexor spasticity or intermittent spasms – a child must have fairly good sitting balance to benefit from such a seat.

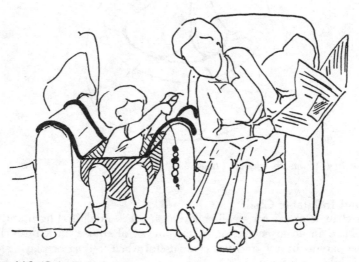

Figure 116. 'Safa' Bath Seat

'Star Rider' Car Seat

The 'Star Rider' car seat, fig. 117 (a), is excellent for most babies and children with little or no head control or sitting balance. The seat is so shaped that it keeps the head and shoulders forward, the harness preventing the child from slipping forwards. The seat, although designed for a car, can be used in the home, it is attached to a chair-back, the wheels on the chair legs making it easy to move around. See fig. 117 (b).

Please note that we do *not recommend* this seat if the child persistently falls to one side or pushes back against the seat and, despite the harness, pushes downwards.

The 'Cosco Go-Go' Seat

The 'Cosco Go-Go' Seat figs. 118 (a) (b), is worth studying for its shape, this chair is washable and can be adjusted to two heights. It has two holes in the back through which a wide band can be placed to secure it to an ordinary chair, useful for example, if you want the child to be at table level. Unfortunately, the firm making this chair has stopped

162

manufacture, the Spastics Society however, are trying to find another manufacturer to produce this type of chair. The Baby Relax Company has now for sale a child's 'T.V.' plastic and steel-framed chair available in red, green and mauve; these can be purchased through the Spastics Society (item 786), and are a good substitute if the 'Cosco Go-Go' Seat cannot be obtained.

When a child is afraid of sitting in a chair without a table in front of him, we have found that this type of seat, when placed in a cardboard box is an excellent way of giving him confidence, and encouraging him to lean forward automatically, as he reaches to pick his toys up off the bottom of the box, or even attempts to reach those that have fallen outside, he feels safe as if necessary he has the sides of the box to hold onto, see fig. 119.

Please note that we do *not recommend* the use of this type of chair unless the child has good sitting balance.

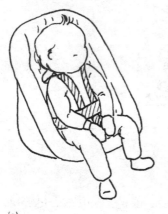

(a)

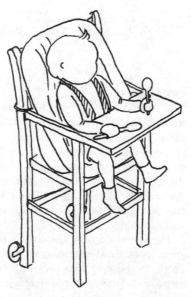

(b)

Figure 117
(a) 'Star Rider' Car Seat
(b) 'Star Rider' Car Seat attached to chair

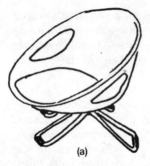
(a)

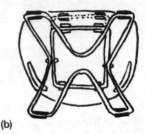
(b)

Figure 118
(a) 'Cosco Go-Go' Seat
(b) Underside showing two height adjustments

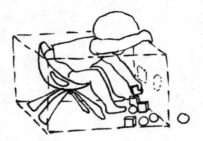

Figure 119. 'Cosco Go-Go' Seat. Inside a cardboard box.

Box Chair

For young children we have recently been using, with considerable success, the box chair with a tray. It is made of wood and is simple to make, see fig. 120 (a). This seat is so designed that the young child can sit with his legs straight out in front of him, a normal position for a young child at this stage of his motor development. The straight back of the box, in combination with the sloping angle of the seat and the narrowness of the sides of the box, gives the child with poor sitting balance, sufficient confidence making additional support or straps unnecessary.

The *correct angle* of the seat is of the utmost importance, as the child's lower back must rest against the support. If the angle of the seat is too steep, the base of the spine will be rounded and when the child reaches forward to play, active extension of the back will be impossible, see fig. 120 (b). If the child's arms have a tendency to press down when he sits, see that the tray is at chest height or tilted. Different trays can be slotted-in to add variety to the child's play.

164

Mothers who have to apply 'jaw control' when feeding the child, sometimes find this seat useful as his sitting balance is fairly adequate it leaves her hands comparatively free. Being small the box has the added advantage that it can be placed on a table at meal-times and at a useful height for the mother.

Please note that we do *not recommend* this chair for the child with poor head control, or those who are floppy or very flexed. A child with asymmetrical patterns of posture and movement may need additional support when sitting in this chair, for example a small sandbag at the hips.

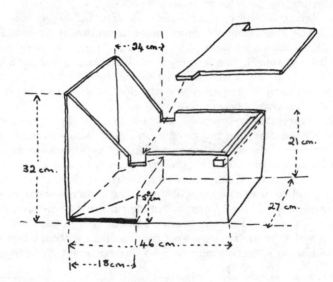

(a)

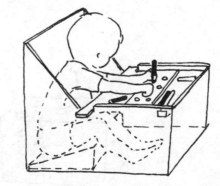

(b)

Figure 120
(a) Box Chair
(b) Box Chair showing example of Tray Fitment

165

Cardboard Boxes for use as chairs

The young child with poor balance will often feel more secure when he sits in a confined space. For this reason we have lately, both for treatment and for play, made use of large cardboard boxes of varying sizes, these can usually be obtained from any large store or supermarket.

A large cardboard box makes an excellent play area as toys can be attached across the top, to the sides, or laid on the floor of the box, or a smaller box can be placed inside to form a table, see fig. 121. It is worth stressing again that sitting need not be a passive or static function, and when the child has reached the stage of moving in the sitting position and is starting to pull himself up to standing and so forth the box makes an excellent practise area for such activities.

When playing in the box, obviously using a far bigger box than illustrated, the child often becomes quite adventurous automatically practising the basic patterns necessary for getting up to standing, having reached this milestone, he starts to try to walk sideways around the inside of the box. It is in fact, a mobile play-pen and being light can be taken into different rooms while mother does the housework without having to worry about her child's safety.

You can vary the make-up of the box to give the child varying sensations. Some days line the bottom and sides with pieces of carpet (display squares of carpets that are no longer in production make an excellent lining and can often be purchases from large stores), squares of soft fluffy-type material, e.g. of which bedroom slippers are made, provide a good contrast. You can also vary the contents of the box, fill it with tissue paper, or newspaper, wrapping up some of his toys, put in odd pieces of foam, odd cartons and varieties of spoons etc.

Please note that we do *not recommend* the use of a cardboard box for a child who has no sitting balance or who has not reached the stage of sitting.

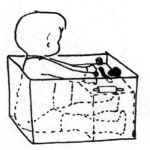

Figure 121. Cardboard Box as play area.

The Cylinder Chair

The cylinder used for this chair is made of thick reinforced cardboard, the cylinders themselves are used commercially. With the section cut-out it forms a useful seat, it can be covered in foam and then with a washable material with a foam cushion added to the seat. The seat is a thick disc of reinforced cardboard and gives the necessary stability to the cylinder, see figs. 122 (a) (b).

This seat has been found most useful at meal-times for children who have fairly good sitting balance, but are still apprehensive when using their hands. The shape of the back of the cylinder keeps the shoulders forward and this makes it easier for the child to use his hands, especially those children who tend to fall back when they lift the spoon to their mouths. The shape gives good support, providing a sense of security for the child. For the young child the seat can be placed on the floor as illustrated, see fig. 122 (c).

Please note that we do *not recommend* this chair unless a child has fairly good sitting balance. Its main function is to enable the child to get better hand function for specific activities while sitting.

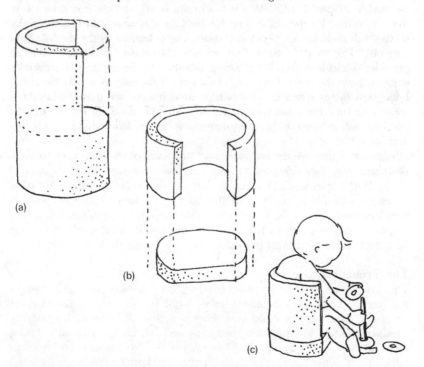

(a)

(b)

(c)

Figure 122
(a) The Cylinder Chair
(b) The Cylinder Chair showing height variations
(c) Child plays in seat which is at floor level.

The Roller Chair

The Roller Chair was designed by the author for the spastic child who has difficulty in sitting and is unable to bend at the hips or to part and bend his legs. Using groin straps, or placing a post between the legs of such a child, which we had previously used, we found for many children to be inadequate – the post kept the knees apart but did not solve the basic problem, i.e. the turning in and pulling of the legs together which takes place at the hips. The roller shape parts the legs high up and makes it easier for the child to bend at his hips and knees and to keep his feet flat on the floor, enabling him to bring his arms forward and to use his hands – the back of the seat is upright and firm, combining well with the padded roller. A design for making the 'Roller Chair' by anyone with an elementary knowledge of carpentry, is shown in fig. 123.

Following the publication of the first edition, I was approached by Mr. M. S. Wason of Church Hill, Totland Bay, Isle of Wight, who wished to produce this chair commercially. Mr. Wason amended my basic design making the height of the back of the seat, the roller and the front handle adjustable, and introducing a form of brake so that the seat could be used at a special table. When the brake is off, the chair can be easily moved around by the child. The Roller Chair is now sold commercially by the 'Educational Supply Association' and is known as the 'Saddle Seat Engine'. The 'Saddle Seat Engine' has the added advantage that it provides a stable object for pushing around the house and is especially enjoyable for the child if another child sits on the seat as a passenger. An important factor when using this type of seat is to see that the height is correct so that the child has his feet flat on the floor, otherwise he will push himself around on his toes, increasing his tendency to stiffen his legs and feet.

Please note that we do *not recommend* this seat, other than as a toy, for the child who has adequate sitting balance – let him sit on a normal chair. If the spastic child when sitting on this type of seat continually flexes his hips lifting his feet off the floor, or is unable to keep both or only one foot flat on the floor, again this chair is *not* suitable. Obviously a child would not benefit from having this seat if he always has his legs bent and wide apart, and has difficulty in keeping them together.

The Triangle Chair

This chair was first designed with either one or two posts attached to the base to keep the legs apart, see figs 124 (a) (b). It is a useful chair for the spastic diplegic child and those athetoid children with spasticity who are inclined to straighten their hips and fall backwards when lifting their arms to use their hands. Designers have also made it more adaptable and in some cases have included various types of tables see figs. 125 – 127. A portable folding canvas corner seat has lately been produced, see fig. 128.

I believe that a type of triangle chair would be useful in the bath for

168

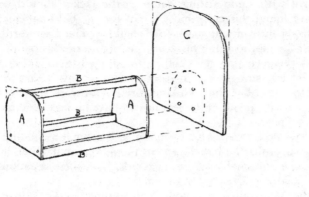

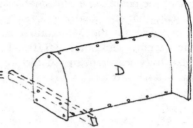

Figure 123. Construction of Roller Chair
A. Cut 2 squares 8″ x 8″, rounded at top, from ½″ plywood.
B. Screw 3 struts between the end pieces, each 13″ long approx. from 1″ x 1″ wood.
C. Chair back made of ¼″ plywood 20″ (high) x 15½″ (wide) rounded at top. Fix A to C with 4 screws.
D. Cut hardboard 14″ x 21½″. Soak overnight in bath, bend over roller frame, and tack into position.
E. Foot-piece (if needed) 1″ x 1″ wood, 16″ long. Screw onto A.

some children, but unfortunately no designer has yet produced it in a material suitable for this purpose.

Please note that we do *not recommend* this type of chair for the child who sits with a very wide base i.e. with a round back and flexed hips and flexed abducted legs, except in cases where the triangle chair is used in a normal chair, see fig. 125 (c) or the adapted model of the chair, see fig. 125 (a) in which the feet can remain flat on the floor, or on a support, see fig. 126.

The 'Mountain' Chair
As this chair, at the time of writing had not been patented by the designer Mr. Mountain, we will refer to the chair by the name used by some therapists. The 'Mountain' chair is made of tubular steel and canvas, with a jacket attached to the top of the back of the chair. The jacket fits over the child's shoulders and chest, an extra band of canvas fitted to the seat of the chair keeps the jacket in place attached to it by 'Velcro', see fig. 129. Immediately the child starts to have improved head

169

and trunk control with some sitting balance, the jacket should be removed. We have found this chair most useful for the older athetoid child who has strong intermittent spasms which throw him backwards, making it difficult for him to bring his arms forward to use his hands.

The chair is so designed that the child is encouraged to sit in 'long sitting' i.e. with his legs straight out in front of him, counteracting the abnormal sitting posture that these children prefer. Later as the child improves, by reducing the depth of the seat he can have his legs bent and his feet flat on the floor.

Please note that we do *not recommend* the use of this chair if a child has such poor head control that he just 'hangs' in the jacket, or if, when he sits in the chair, he is still unable to use his hands, both these situations indicate that the child is not ready for sitting.

Enquiries for the 'Mountain' chair should be sent direct to the designer Mr. Jeremy Mountain of 110, Muirfield Road, Worthing, Sussex. The following measurements should be given – shoulder to bottom; hips to knees; knees to feet.

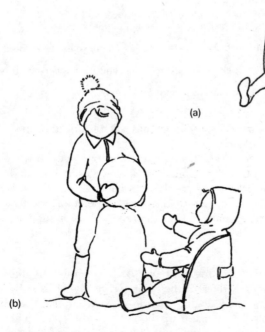

(a)

(b)

Figure 124
(a) Triangle Chair
(b) Making use of a triangle chair outside

170

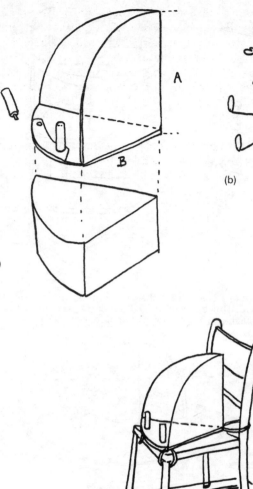

(a)

(b)

(c)

Figure 125
(a) Modifications of the triangle chair. An extra wooden base can be clipped on to enable the child to sit with his legs bent and feet flat on the floor.
(b) When measuring take shoulders to base, see A, and for base to knee, see B, and allow 6″ – 8″ for angle.
(c) The principle of the triangle chair adapted to the seat of an ordinary chair, using just the side pieces and two posts. Skids are optional. Chair can be moved from room to room, from chair to floor, to the car, or used when visiting other people's houses.

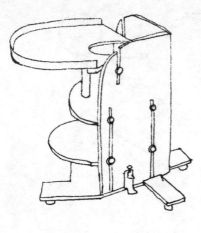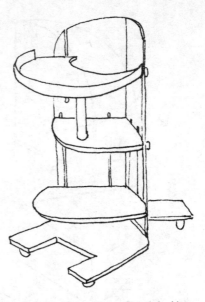

Figure 126. This fully adjustable corner seat chair is designed by Mr. J.A. Ling and made by him at 'J. & C. Office furniture', 1, Barbon Close, Great Ormond · Street, London, W.C.1. Available in larger sizes if required.

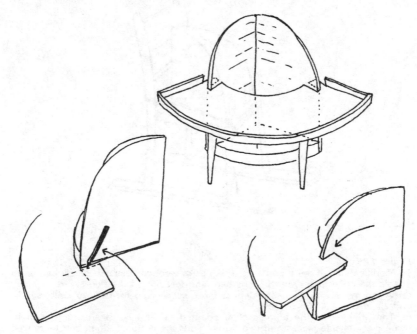

Figure 127. Triangle Chair with cut-out table attachment. For correct angle for table cut-out place a triangle chair on table top, allow 3'' cut-out for stability.

172

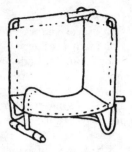

Figure 128. Folding Canvas Corner Seat. Suitable for 2 – 8 year age group. Folds flat to 26'' x 18¾''. Provides secure seating for small children with sitting problems, especially *spastic* children, no strapping needed; developed at The Centre for Spastic Children, London. Enquiries to:-
Temple Engineering Co.
P.O. Box No.1,
High Street, Cowes,
Isle of Wight.

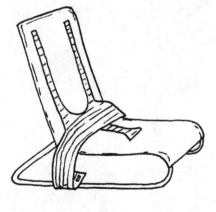

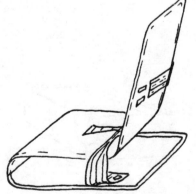

Figure 129. The 'Mountain' chair for the more severely handicapped *athetoid* child.

Foam shapes or Packing Cases

There are now available a variety of shapes and sizes of cut-out foam produced by manufacturers of foam products.

Fig. 130 illustrates how a chair can be made from the type of packing case or foam which is firm and easy to cut. Ask at your local radio shop as some of their products may be delivered in this type of case; thick foam rubber can be used as an alternative. When the child sits on the floor a wooden or cardboard box can be used as a modified table in conjunction with the packing case. Fig. 131 illustrates the use of this type of box as a table fitment with a bar on which to hang toys for the athetoid child.

Please note that we do *not recommend* the use of foam shapes for inactive, passive or floppy children, as they will just relax against the foam.

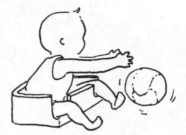

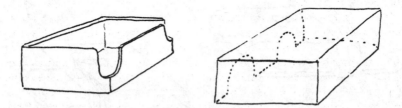

Figure 130. A small packing case (e.g. as used for wireless sets), adapted as a seat for a young child. If the legs are stiff and tend to cross, cut out the part as illustrated, using a razor blade. If the legs are *floppy* and turn out excessively the cut-out should be modified.

These seats can be placed on an easy chair or sofa, as well as on the floor or in a car. They are very light and useful to carry the child around the house in. If the material is 'scratchy' make a pillow case of towelling and slip it inside.

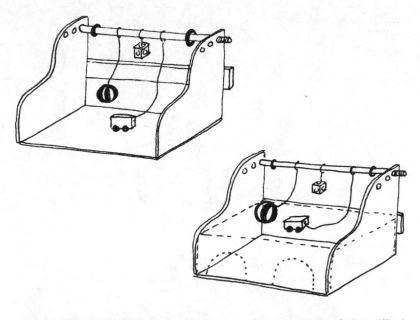

Figure 131. Adjustable frame for hanging toys. *Athetoid* children find it difficult to handle their toys, which frequently 'fly away' from them. Where a tray with a deep side is not adequate, we have found that attaching the toys to a bar is useful. The idea illustrated was made by a parent for his daughter, an *athetoid* child, to play sitting on the floor. The sides are wood, the base hardboard, a piece of wood at the back joins the sides to make them more secure. Having three holes at the top of each side enables the bar to be placed near or far away from the child, as required. The case acts as a table if required, this can be modified to fit onto a table for a bigger child.

Chairs and tables for the Older Cerebral Palsied Child

While on the subject of sitting, it is necessary to refer to tables and their use in conjunction with chairs. Figs. 134 to 135 show a 'cut-out' table used in conjunction with a roller.

The distance between the child's chair and the table varies in accordance with the child's handicap, the usual space being roughly two inches. For the athetoid child, a table at just above knee level, with the chair slightly away from the table, will help to counteract his tendency to fall backwards. On the other hand, the spastic child will manage better if the table is higher in relation to the chair, this will help to inhibit his tendency to lean on the table, pushing down with his arms and shoulders, making it impossible for him to reach forward with his arms. In the case of the ataxic child, the table should be even higher in relation to the chair, enabling him to steady his arms making co-ordination of his hand movements easier, until he has learned to time, grade, and direct his movements himself. Fig. 136 illustrates a solid wooden chair and table for the more severely affected child with no sitting balance.

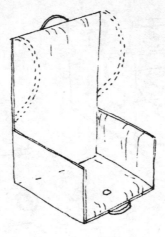

Figure 132. A portable chair for the older child – can be used in a wheel chair, car-seat or kitchen chair. Loops can be attached to the front of the seat and top of the back and pommel, or groin straps can be attached to the hole in the seat.

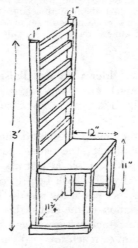

Figure 133. The 'Pëto' chair designed at the Pëto Institute, Budapest, Hungary. This is a solid chair, which can also be used by the child to push when he starts to walk, by extending the bars which join the legs, thus forming a type of ski. For easy construction the chair base can be made out of a solid box.

176

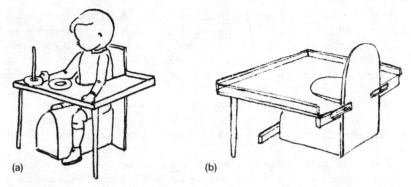

(a)   (b)

Figure 134
(a) Child sitting on roller chair with cut-out table in front. Note that height of roller is level with the knees. There should be a space of about 2″ between the child and table at the front and at the sides.
(b) Cut-out table showing the use of door bolts to attach table to the chair-back.

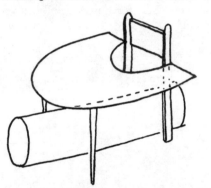

Figure 135. Chair-back with cut-out table, placed over ordinary roller for use when the child has some sitting balance, permitting sideways movement of the child while sitting.

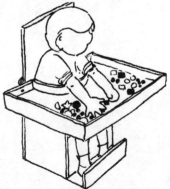

Figure 136. A solid wooden chair, with cut-out table and a wooden guard foot-stop.

177

Despite what we have said about adaptable chairs, the relation of tables to the chairs, and the fact that they may be comfortable or convenient and so on, we must stress that the aim must be to reach the stage when the child can sit at a table completely unsupported, without adjustments to his chair or for the need of a table to be placed in front of him.

Watch the child's posture closely when he is sitting and be prepared to make adjustments to the chair, it is unwise to postpone making adjustments merely on the grounds that he may need an entirely new chair in a few months' time.

Finally we must emphasise that *your aim* must be to get your child to sit on *an ordinary chair* as soon as he has started to get some sitting balance, and treatment will be directed towards helping your child to get sitting balance, he must practise this ability and obviously will not be able to do so if supported everywhere. Complete independence will only be achieved when the child has sufficient balance to use both hands for skilled activities, can get his chair for himself, pull it up to the table and get on and off by himself.

Chapter 13

HAMMOCKS, WEDGES AND PRONE BOARDS

HAMMOCKS

A hammock is useful for the severely affected small child who is very stiff when lying on his back as he is unable to lift or turn his head and cannot be left on his own when lying on his tummy.

Since publication of the first edition many firms are advertising hammocks for use by the baby in the car. Hammocks are usually made of netting material therefore we suggest that you put a cover inside the hammock, as the hands of the cerebral palsied child can easily become entangled in the mesh, or even better buy one made of sail-cloth or canvas. Hammocks can be suspended between the uprights of a door frame, or between two trees or supports in the garden, at about two or three feet from the ground, figs. 137 (a) (b), or suspended between the uprights of the cot, fig. 137(c). Fig. 138, shows a design for a hammock than can be made at home, in sail-cloth or deckchair canvas.

Apart from the pleasure it gives the child, the advantages of a hammock are – it supports the child's shoulders bringing them forward, preventing the head from pushing back, the gentle sideways movement also tends to bring the head into mid-line with the body. A hammock is soft and moulds itself to the shape of the child's body, whereas lying on any flat hard surface causes the child to push back and reinforces his spasms. As an alternative for the young child a thick piece of foam can be cut out to provide the same 'shape' as a hammock, see fig. 139.

As the child gradually gets used to being in a hammock he starts to bring his hands together and to put them to his mouth. Very often for the first time he sees his feet, and realises they are part of himself, making attempts to reach them and bring them to his mouth. By swinging the hammock in different directions the child can be encouraged to roll, kick, sit up, play with a toy and so on – a good opportunity to combine play with treatment. As with any other position, the child should not remain in a hammock for too long, say – no more than three quarters of an hour at a time.

BOUNCING CRADLE

For the young baby with the type of abnormal patterns mentioned in the paragraphs on hammocks, we have found that the 'Bouncing Cradle' – see fig. 140, fulfils the same purpose for the baby as the hammock does for the older child. If the baby should start to kick with stiff legs that have a tendency to cross, try raising the buttocks by putting a small pad underneath, sometimes extra padding around the strap between the legs will also prevent the crossing of the legs.

Please note that we do *not recommend* the use of the 'Bouncing Cradle' if the child still remains asymmetrical and continues to kick abnormally whilst he is in it.

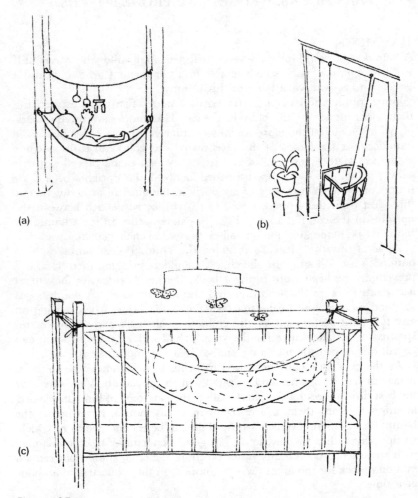

Figure 137
(a) While you are working in the kitchen, instead of allowing the more severely affected child to lie on the floor, a useful alternative is to let him swing on a hammock slung between the door-posts.
(b) For the older less severely affected child a swing can be hung from the lintel of the door-posts.
(c) When the baby is resting during the *daytime* and you are about, a hammock can be slung between the uprights of the baby's cot.

180

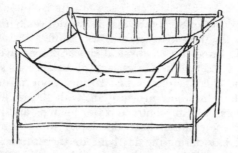

Figure 138. Design for a hammock that can be made at home. A thick reinforced cotton or sailcloth is the most suitable material. When necessary, extra pockets can be made for pillows to put behind the head and under the knees to prevent the child from slipping down. The hammock can be made rigid – to keep the sides apart – by inserting wood rods into pleats at the top and bottom.

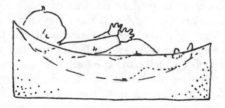

Figure 139. Foam section, cut out to provide a hammock shape.

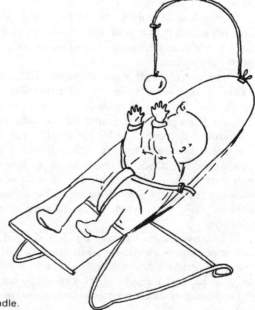

Figure 140. The Bouncing Cradle.

WEDGES

There are children who for many reasons are not really ready to sit in a chair but do so for the convenience of the family, e.g. at mealtimes or when mother is busy. Their physical development may be delayed, complete lack of head control and lack of balance in sitting may, in effect, make the child helpless when sitting, poor posture making it impossible for him to adjust his position, with the result that he is in danger of developing flexor contractures at his hips and knees.

As soon as these children have developed some head control they should spend periods during the day lying on their tummies. Why do we suggest this position? If you place your child on his tummy you will notice immediately how much more symmetrical he is, how he is now able to lift his head and, at the same time, to straighten his back, this in turn facilitates the straightening of his hips and legs, minimising a tendency for the legs to cross and come together. If you have ever lain on your tummy when, for example, sunbathing you will appreciate how tiring it is if you now try to read, in no time the back of your neck, your back and often your arms tire quickly, but if you place something under your chest or lie at a slight angle the position is much easier to maintain.

As our aim is to get the child to reach forward and use his hands we must provide a support which can be adjusted to suit his needs, while at the same time inhibiting abnormal patterns of posture and movement developing. Wedges can be made from foam, canvas, inflatables, or wood with a layer of foam and a cover of washable material. There are firms that will spray the foam with a material that makes them waterproof and much easier to clean.

The following points should be noted when deciding on a wedge, bearing in mind that your aim is always to get the child playing on his tummy with *minimal support,* leading as soon as possible to him playing sitting on a chair.

There are children who, to begin with, need a wedge with a steep incline, if so it is *most important* that the play area be raised, see figs. 141 (a) (b) (c). *Too often the value of a wedge is lost* by having the play area too low, far from helping the child this actually *increases* his flexor spasticity. The child will manage to lift his head but at the same time his shoulders will press down and turn in, this will make it difficult or impossible for him to use his hands. If the child is asymmetrical the use of a sandbag will correct this, place it along the side of the trunk and under the shoulder, or by the side of the hips. *Never* place a sandbag on the child's bottom while he is lying on his tummy as this will increase his flexor spasticity.

It is advisable to see that the feet do not become stiff and pointed; whenever you pass by, or while playing with your child, spend a few minutes bending his ankles, i.e. his feet up, while at the same time keeping his legs turned out, also check to see that his hips are not stiff.

Continual re-assessment is necessary to see if any adjustments to the

182

wedge, or extra support when used, are still needed, or in fact whether the child still even needs a wedge.

See figs. 142 and 143 (a) (b) for types of supports and wedges. Fig. 144 (a) (b) illustrates an *adjustable* wedge recently designed by Dr. D. Mills the designer of the mini-prone board.

(a)

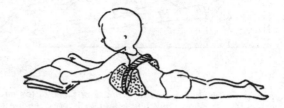

(b)

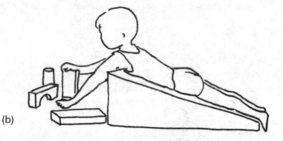

(c)

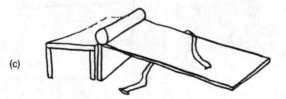

Figure 141
Various ways of enabling a child to play while lying on his tummy. Note that the hips and legs are left free, it is important that the child is able to move in this position.
(a) A bolster, with webbing support for the child who rolls over immediately he is placed on his tummy.
(b) A foam wedge; the child in the illustration does *not* push down from his shoulders and can therefore manage to play on the floor.
(c) A variation of the padded sloping board, including safety straps for the child who *does* push down at the shoulders. The small roller helps to keep the child's shoulders forward and up. The stool or box should be varied in height according to the needs of the child.

183

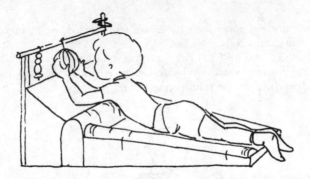

Figure 142
Another adaptation of the sloping board. A board or piece of foam-rubber cut into a wedge long enough to allow the child's feet to hang over the edge, as illustrated. The sides are built up leaving room for the child to move but preventing him from falling off, a roll is placed in the front. As some children find it difficult to lift and bend their arms when lying on their tummies, we have sloped the top of the playing area.

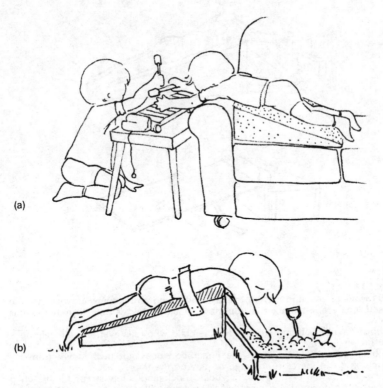

(a)

(b)

Figure 143
Two uses of a wedge to encourage reaching out while playing.

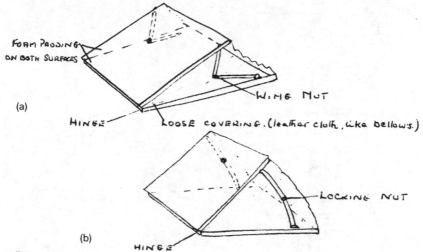

Figure 144

(a) The idea of the adjustable wedge is to provide height adjustment, the variation of the angle of the wedge illustrated is from 0° to 90°. The wedge is made of wood, padded and covered in a washable material. Although not shown it would be advisable to fix a cone-shaped piece of wood to the top side of the wedge to prevent the child from slipping down as the angle is widened.

(b) An alternative design giving less variation of angle say, from 25° to 50° or 30° to 60°. Two overlapping triangle boxes hinged at the narrow end with matching grooves cut in the side, to allow a locking-nut to fix the angle. The advantage being that the wedge can be padded on all five sides and therefore is more rigid. A slot can be made at each side for a body-strap if required.

PRONE BOARDS

School children spend a number of hours at a table or desk, this sometimes presents a problem for the child whose overall pattern is one of flexion. In this case prolonged time spent in sitting can lead to flexor contractures developing at hips and knees, and in the case of some children their asymmetrical sitting posture often affects their eye-hand co-ordination. Some schools provide such children with a prone board to use in the classrooms and in the dining room.

The advantages of the prone board for a flexed *asy*mmetrical child is that it provides *sym*metry, and prevents the shoulder girdle from pressing down, so that the child can reach forward and use his hands. His hips and knees are kept extended and apart and his feet dorsi-flexed and any tendency of the feet to turn in or turn out can be controlled.

Numerous designs of the prone board have been made, making them as adaptable as possible – each board being tailored to the child's individual needs – see figs. 145 (a) (b) (c) 146 and 147 illustrating the Glenrosa prone board used at the Glenrose School, Canada. Any additional support needed, for example, straps across the thighs or knees should be as few as possible and carefully placed. The child should never rest or hang over the top of the board and should be so placed that he can extend actively while he uses his hands.

185

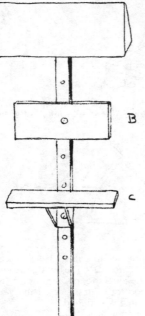

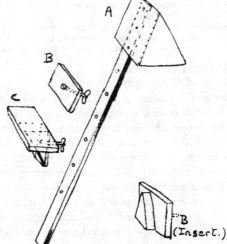

Figure 145
Glenrosa Prone Board
A. chest-piece, padded.
B. knee-board, padded.
   Can be fitted with an abduction wedge, see insert.
C. Foot board.
All fixtures are adjustable, by using bolts and wing-nuts through holes in upright.
Length of upright depends on angle required and position i.e. at table, sink, etc.
(4'' x 2'' wood)
Chest-piece 8'' deep, length must go 6'' beyond arms on either side. Knee board
8'' deep, 14'' wide.

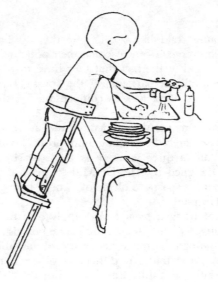

Figure 146
Helping at home using the Glenrosa prone board while standing on the board.

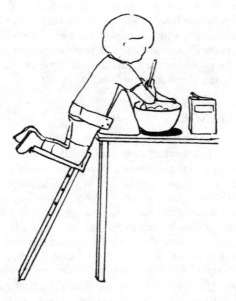

Figure 147
Helping at home using the Glenrosa prone board while kneeling on the board.

Mini-Prone Board

There are some young children who, despite their ability to use their hands for play, are prevented from reaching their potential owing to their poor sitting balance, and to the fact that they have to rely on one hand for support. Some of them, particularly the spastic diplegic children, resort to sitting between their legs to compensate for their inadequate sitting balance.

In an attempt to overcome this difficulty, and as an alternative to a special chair, we have lately been using mini-prone boards for the age group two and a half to three years. Figs. 148 (a) (b) (c) illustrate a mini-prone board designed by Dr. D. Mills a general practitioner of Surrey, whose patient, a spastic diplegic of two, is being treated by me at Charing Cross Hospital.

The advantages of using a *prone* board apply also to the *mini*-prone board. It is hoped that by using these mini-prone boards at an early age, that the child will be able to make better use of his ability to acquire more advanced skills, and that any difficulties of eye-hand control and specific problems relating to future learning can be dealt with earlier; the child also enjoys a new view of his environment, and of the people and activities around him – all essential adjuncts to learning.

When general control in combination with jaw control is necessary, feeding some two-year olds can become a problem and mothers with more severely affected children have found the mini-prone board a help. For some children the first steps towards self feeding will be easier if the child is on a mini-prone board. For both mother and child the mini-prone board provides yet another means by which the child can join in and observe his mother's activities as she moves around; as the board is adjustable it can be placed against the kitchen table as his mother cooks, or near the sink when she washes up and so on.

OUTSIDE APPLIANCES

In the Neuro-Developmental approach to treatment of cerebral palsied children, we do not use what can broadly be described as 'outside' appliances, for example, calipers, other than occasionally for the older age group. Therefore I do not propose to deal with these appliances, with the exception of the 'Gaiter' splint which we recommend, on occasions, as an aid to standing for some children to encourage extension of the legs, see fig. 149 (a) (b). A decision to use them can *only* be made by your child's therapist, she will tell you that they should be used for only a limited time for standing, and should not be used for walking as they 'fix' the knees in extension and walking in them would only lead to the child developing an abnormal gait. A smaller type of the 'Gaiter' splint has been found useful for keeping the elbows of the athetoid child straight; again we must remind you that a decision to use such a splint should be made only by your therapist.

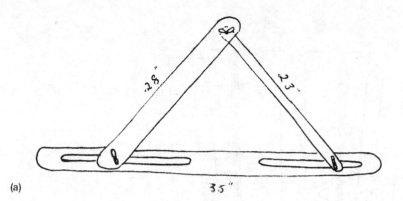

(a)

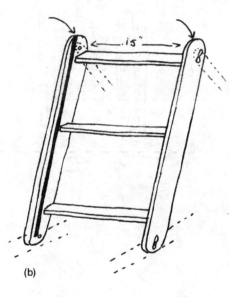

(b)

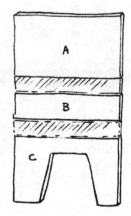

(c)

Figure 148
The adjustable mini-prone board provides a number of different angles for the child, i.e. between lying and standing, the adjustment is made possible by moving the wing-nut. The frame is made of wood. Angle iron (with prepared holes in it) could also be used.
(a) Side view, showing wing-nuts for adjustment of angle.
(b) Front view, with slot for sliding in chest, hip and leg boards (arrowed).
(c) Sliding boards A. chest B. hips C. legs. With narrow 'fill-in' boards between.

189

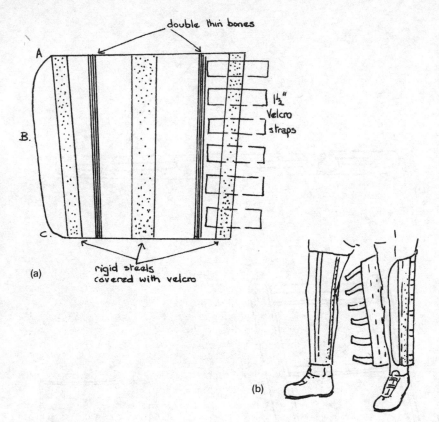

Figure 149
(a) Design for 'gaiter' splint.
(b) Correct method for application of 'gaiter' splint.

Chapter 14

AIDS TO MOBILITY

Between the ages of twelve to eighteen months a child continues to learn as he explores his environment. He finds his way into cupboards, pulling open and shutting doors, inspecting and experimenting with and promptly discarding the contents; no place in the house being left undisturbed.

Owing to their lack of mobility this period of exploration is one that many cerebral palsied children unfortunately are compelled, to a large extent, to forego. It is therefore important that we should make full use of the many aids that are available, many of which are designed to assist a handicapped child to move around as independently as possible.

We should encourage the child, as frequently as practicable, through-out the day, to accustom himself to the use of these aids and not merely as the result of a directive from us.

Figs. 150 to 163 illustrate a number of the means by which the child can be mobile both inside and outside the home, in the latter case, of course, more supervision will be needed to begin with.

The items shown are generally of use to the one to five age group. It must be appreciated that some of the ideas illustrated, for example bicycles and a motor car, are just the ordinary type of toy used by *normal* children; that fact in itself makes their use by handicapped children more desirable and attractive. The more *'ordinary'* the things that the handicapped child can use, to encourage a sense of not being *'different'* from his companions, the greater will be his confidence and pleasure in his achievement.

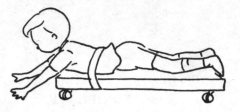

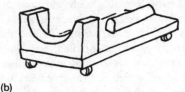

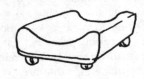

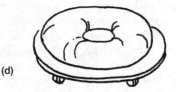

Figure 150
(a) For the young *spastic diplegic* child who normally creeps on the floor. A simple wooden board 2'' thick with four 'Shepherds' castors; this will encourage the child to move around, pushing with straight arms. For the very young child whose legs are not stiff the only support he may need is a band around his body, as illustrated. Where further support is required a harness can be made to deal with the child's specific problems.
(b) This modification of the board is for the more severely handicapped child. The front is raised to make it easier for the child to lift his head and his back and help him to get his arms straight, it can be made of foam-rubber or half of a wireless set or similar type packing case. A roll made of foam-rubber can be fixed to the rear part of the board and will help to keep the legs apart. In more severe cases a separate wood frame section may be necessary.
(c) A small scooped-out stool with 'Shepherd's' castors for the child who has *'weak'* rather than *spastic* legs to encourage him to use them and not his arms to push himself around.
(d) Modification of the stool; a padded wheel with rubber tyre. These can be bought from most stores.

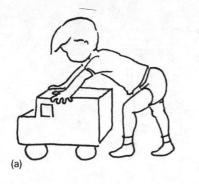
(a)

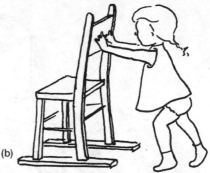
(b)

Figure 151
To walk our weight must be forward; a problem for many cerebral palsied children.

(a) and (b) illustrate how by varying the height and weight of the object pushed we can also vary the amount of hip flexion. The child can progress to pushing a chair with rungs see 'Pëto' chair.

For the child who has begun to walk but who lacks sufficient balance to do so without support, we have recently tried attaching a broom handle in an upright position on each side of an ordinary chair-back. This provides a simple form of 'walker' as the weight of the chair means that the child has to bring his weight forward as he pushes the chair along.

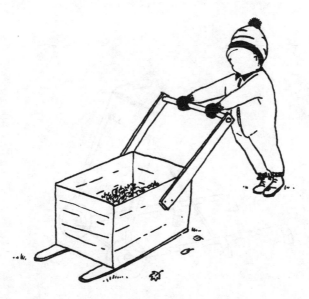

Figure 152. A large wooden box makes a good home-walker, the additional stability will give resistance and make it easier for the *athetoid* and *ataxic* child to push. Wooden skids can be added to make it simpler to push over carpets.

193

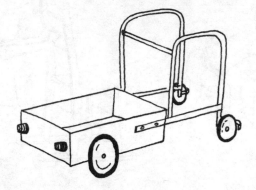

Figure 153. This baby-walker can be purchased from The Educational Supply Association; the frame gives it added weight and security. The child can progress from holding the horizontal bar to the side bars.

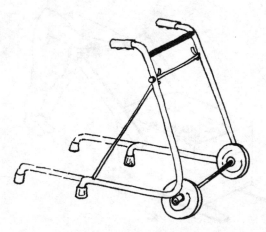

Figure 154. The 'Adjustable Rolator Walker' – Kiddies model made by Carters Ltd. is a satisfactory walker for cerebral palsied children, if required one can now purchase it with the 'Cheyne Walk Bar', as illustrated, height 20'' - 25'' handgrip to floor; 25'' - 30'' handgrip to floor.

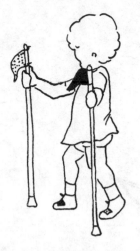

Figure 155. Two poles with rubber tips are ideal for the child who has some standing balance and is starting to walk on her own. While they provide some support she will be unable to lean on them and therefore has to work to remain upright.

Start by holding the top of the sticks, but as soon as possible, let the child manage on her own.

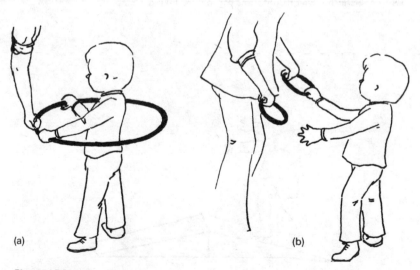

(a) (b)

Figure 156
Hoops and quoit rings make a useful stable and mobile support, bridging the gap from being held when walking to independent walking.
(a) A hoop gives the most support.
(b) The child first learns to grasp the quoit rings in *pronation* as illustrated, but should progress as soon as possible to grasping them in *supination* as this will help to inhibit any flexor spasticity which causes the pulling down of the arms. Finally the child walks holding both quoit rings himself.

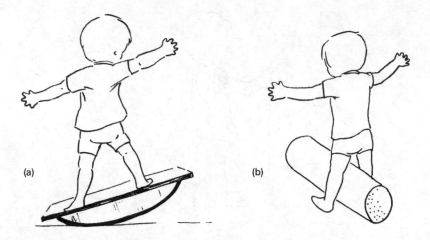

Figure 157
(a) To stand and walk we must be able to balance. To take a step we need to transfer our weight from one leg to the other. The balance-board illustrated is a good way of getting the child to learn to do this.
For the small child a home-made balance-board can be made by nailing a large rolling pin to a piece of wood.
(b) By walking with a foot on each side of a roller placed on the ground the child has to transfer his weight onto one leg before taking a step.

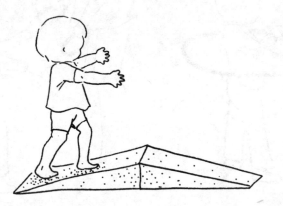

Figure 158. Walking on foam wedges placed in this way is fun as well as a learning situation. The child has to adjust his position to the incline, and the softness of the foam facilitates movements of the feet (balance reactions). Vary the speed, direction of walking, i.e. forwards, backwards, or sideways, finally get the child to stop on command – to begin with the child could have a pole in each hand for support to give him confidence.

196

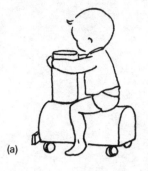

(a)

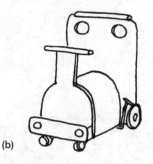

(b)

Figure 159
(a) For the child who has good arms and moves around the floor by 'bunny-hopping' and is not old enough to ride a tricycle; this is a modification of the 'Roller Seat'. The child has to move his legs to push himself around, the roller helps to keep them apart and turned out. The funnel keeps the arms up and apart.
(b) The Engine Seat designed by Mr. M.S. Wason.

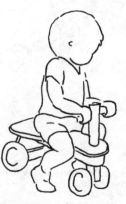

Figure 160. 'Galt's' wooden tricycle, without pedals. We have found this the most stable first tricycle.

197

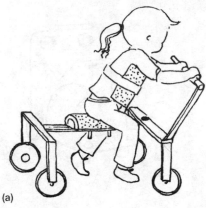

(a)

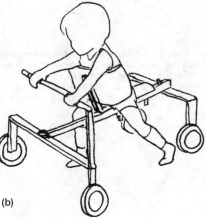

(b)

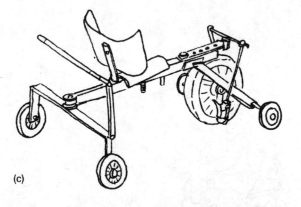

(c)

Figure 161
(a) and (b) The Spider Walker. C.P. Steerable Walker *without* pedals for the younger or more severely affected child.
(c) The C.P. Tricycle Mk. 2 *with* pedals.
   NOTE: Fig. 161 (a) (b) and (c) have been designed by The Ontario Crippled Children's Centre, 350, Rumsey Road, Postal Station R, Toronto 17, Ontario, Canada.

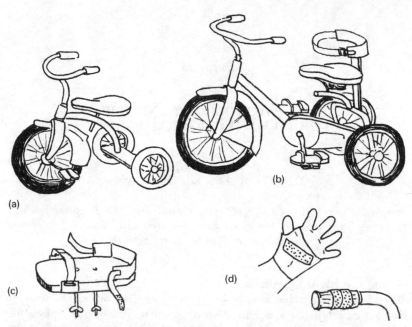

Figure 162
(a) A tricycle with pedal attachment to the front wheel, suitable for young children.
(b) Tricycle with chain drive and independent steering for the older child, back support to seat.
(c) Foot attachment for pedals. The base is made of wood with metal strip around the heel, webbing straps with 'Velcro' fastenings. Two bolts with wing-nuts are used to hold the foot attachment firmly to the pedals. For some less handicapped children an old gym shoe or baseball shoe can be attached to the pedals.
(d) Bands of 'Velcro' attached to the palm of the child's mitten. Two 'Velcro' strips attached to the handle bars as illustrated give the child extra confidence.

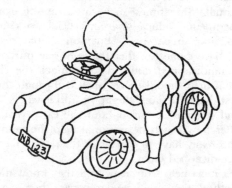

Figure 163. A car *without* pedals is an excellent way of encouraging a child to get around who is apprehensive about moving on his own. A car *with pedals*, as illustrated, can be recommended as a good way of encouraging mobility in the *ataxic, hemiplegic* or *mildly affected* child.

Chapter 15

THE PSYCHOLOGIST AND THE
CHILD WITH CEREBRAL PALSY

By Mary Gardner
B.Sc. (Econ), Dip. Ed., Dip. Psych.

Principal Psychologist, Charing Cross Hospital and The Hospital for Sick Children, Great Ormond Street, London, also previously visiting Educational Psychologist to Spastic Society Schools.

Asking the Right Questions

If a young child is handicapped, it is natural that we should want to find out exactly what is holding him up, so that we can make plans for helping him, and seeing how far and in what ways we can reduce the difficulties. In the case of children with severe cerebral palsy, this process of finding out what is wrong can be quite complicated. This is because spasticity and other forms of cerebral palsy are due to some impairment in part of the brain. Since the brain is very complex, and controls most of our behaviour and learning, our speech, motor movements, our thinking and feeling etc. it is no simple matter to sort these things out, and to find out what is causing the difficulties, and then to present a remedy. The joint efforts of experts working in close partnership with parents are essential. Sometimes such an array of experts (medical, psychological, therapeutic, educational and social work, to name a few) seems very formidable to parents – but you should realize that these experts exist and have come together for only one purpose; to help the family and the handicapped child. The younger the child, the more important it is that help should be channelled through the parents; they are the child's first diagnosticians, therapists and teachers. Their influence is paramount and remains so throughout the early years of the child's life, and no matter how much professional help the family is getting, it is the parents who really have to cope with the day-to-day problems that arise with any handicapped child.

Parents can get most help from experts if they know more about their work, and the methods they use. The parents are then in a better position to ask the right questions. You should always ask questions without constantly worrying whether your queries might be viewed as criticism. Most experts really like answering questions, as this reassures them of the importance of their work and helps to reduce their tendency to look at problems purely from the point of view of their own expertise.

In this chapter we will deal with the work of one of these experts – the child psychologist and his or her part in helping the parents and the child with a handicap.

How Children Learn

The psychologist's main interest is how children learn. The more you know about how children learn, the better chance you have of helping a child who has difficulties in learning. Children learn because:

They want to – all children have an inborn wish to explore their surroundings, to seek new experience. It is extremely rare to find a child so handicapped that he cannot demonstrate his eagerness to learn. Children also need to have the confidence necessary for learning, and this is something parents can influence.

They have the basic physical and mental equipment that is necessary for learning:

   Their various senses, eyes, hands, ears, through which to take in information.

   The brain to attend, to perceive, to organise and make sense out of what they have taken in through their senses, to remember certain things, and to store these for future use.

   The basic equipment to give out or to communicate a response – through their voice or their hands and bodily movements.

They live in a stimulating environment – which offers experience, new information, in digestible and repeatable forms.

Babies start learning right from birth; for example a small baby (or any young creature) makes a variety of unco-ordinated movements. By chance, some of these result in a sensation that he finds enjoyable. The baby's waving arms, while he is lying in his pram, may, for instance, encounter a dangling ring, which he may hold on to by an automatic reflex grasp. His reactions are too primitive and disorganised to grip the ring intentionally, but gradually over days and weeks of repeating this same movement, the developing brain discerns a pattern which finally results (by around six months) in the baby being instantly able to grasp the ring whenever it is in view. From this example, we can see that a baby learns, by means of repetition, to co-ordinate hand and eye movements.

In more complex situations, repetition and practice may be just as important. We have all observed and wondered at the apparently purposeless dropping of toys over the side of a high-chair or pram. When the child repeatedly cries for the toy to be picked up, we might be justified in thinking that he is doing it merely to annoy. This may be so in an older child, but in a young baby who has recently learnt to sit up, the action shows that he is beginning to have a glimmering that objects continue to exist, even though they have disappeared from sight. This is such a novel and fascinating idea to the child, that he feels the need to drop the toy over and over again to see if the same thing happens each time. By means of these simple actions, he is beginning to appreciate quite complicated ideas of cause and effect, and the influence of gravity, of which he needs to be aware before tackling more advanced activities, such as climbing or building with bricks.

A psychologist once tried a simple experiment with his infant son to see how many times he would repeat a 'peep-bo' game before losing interest. He never found out – the father's interest was exhausted by the hundredth time, but he reported that his son showed as much surprise and delight on seeing his father's face reappear over the blanket on the final occasion, as on the first.

A baby also learns about the world by experimenting and trying things out for himself. Telling a child constantly "not to touch" is depriving him of a necessary sensory experience in the same way as shutting him in a darkened room. The child learns about the characteristics of things around him by comparing what his eyes and ears tell him with what he can feel with his hands and mouth.

Another important way that a child learns is by imitation. The earliest imitative behaviour is connected with making sounds. A baby babbles spontaneously during the earliest months, but by about twelve months, many babies will attempt to make the same sounds as the adult who is playing with him. When he is alone in his cot, he practises these sounds, listening to himself doing so and gradually widening his repertoire. A recent study has shown that babies by the age of eighteen months are beginning to 'specialise' when they babble in those sounds which are most common in their native language; we can see from this that imitation starts very early in a child's life.

These simple examples show the way in which babies begin to make sense out of the mass of impressions that bombard them from all sides; making sense out of the sounds and sights and the feel of things around them; moving, and manipulating things, vocalising and talking and generally getting an increased degree of understanding and control of their surroundings.

How does a child with severe cerebral palsy learn?

Learning In The Handicapped Child
The fundamentals for effective learning are the same for the handicapped as for all children, with, of course, some differences of emphasis and timing when the handicaps are severe.

When we were considering the learning processes important to children, we noted that learning involves: *Eagerness and confidence* – they strive to achieve – they have inner drives to explore and to seek new experiences, and they also possess the confidence to do so.

Confidence is very important for learning. Although the drive and eagerness to learn may not be so clearly evident in some very severely handicapped children, for the vast majority the urge to learn is there; but it may be reduced by frustration and failure. This is likely to occur when the stimulation given to a child and the activities expected of him are either too difficult and upsetting, or, at the other extreme, too simple and boring – both of which provide the child with little or no sense of achievement. He may therefore fail to develop a view of himself as a competent and managing person.

Confidence is increased by parents' encouragement and praise for what their child does correctly – rather than by constantly drawing attention to his inadequacies.

Sometimes a child's failures are not really failures but simply a matter of the parents setting standards that are too high. Parents' *expectations* about their child's rate of learning are very important. These expectations must be realistic, and the standards they expect their child to reach in walking, handling things, using speech and reasoning things out, must be related to the severity of the child's handicap – physically, intellectually and emotionally, and it is here that the help of the professional team can be useful, in setting reasonable expectations and reasonable targets. Otherwise parents may be expecting either too much or too little of their child, he may become discouraged and show less eagerness to learn and have less confidence about doing so.

Basic Mental And Physical Equipment For Learning

A cerebral palsied child's difficulties in controlling his movements will, in some situations tend to slow up his learning. As Nancie Finnie has shown in the main body of this book, a baby, particularly during his first two years of life, learns a great deal through his hands and bodily sensations and through his movements in relation to persons and objects in his surroundings. The ways of handling and types of equipment that she suggests are of help, not only in improving the child's practical activities, such as in feeding, or dressing, but in the development of his ideas of space, form and distance and those other concepts that are necessary for him to organise the mass of impressions that he is receiving from the outside world. This brings us to one of the main contributions of the psychologist in finding out about how children learn; that is, the measurement of abilities.

The Measurement Of Intelligence

Intelligence is the ability to learn, to reason things out and to profit from experience. People differ in their intelligence, from the very bright to the very dull, and these differences between people are due to three factors:

> The kind of brain they have at birth, and the quantity and quality of the nerve cells and their connections
>
> Whether or not there has been any impairment or damage to the nerve cells, and if so, what parts of the brain have been affected
>
> Factors outside the child – his family life and the stimulation and encouragement it offers.

203

Now the second of these three factors is obviously important in the case of children with cerebral palsy. Some of the brain cells originally present, have been impaired in some way, such as by the lack of oxygen at birth, and this cannot be directly repaired, but its effects can be overcome, to some extent, by training. In some children the impairment to the nerve cells in the brain becomes evident during the first year of life, usually because the child's motor control is affected and he fails to sit up or move around at the expected time. In other children both the child's motor control and his reasoning abilities are affected, either to a greater or lesser degree.

How Do We Measure Intelligence In The Young Child?

Parents, quite naturally, when looking at signs of their child's progress, compare him with his brothers and sisters or with friends' children, making allowances for differences in ages, and noting how 'quick on the uptake' certain children are, compared with others, in their daily life, and in their play with bricks, toys, words, books, etc. The psychologist makes the same sort of comparison, only in a more systematic way, and with the help of intelligence tests that have been carefully worked out over many decades. These tests give us a fairly accurate idea of what abilities are to be expected of the average one year old, two year old, three year old and so on. For example, if a child aged two, completes the set of little problems which are suitable for a two year old, such as building with bricks, scribbling with a pencil, naming a certain number of toys and a few pictures, picking out a particular toy on request, etc., we can say that this child has a mental age (M.A.) of two years. Since this mental age corresponds exactly with his actual age (A.A.) of two years, we can say that he is of normal intelligence. Another way of expressing this is to say that he has an IQ of 100.

The IQ figure is simply a convenient way of expressing the degree to which the mental age corresponds to the actual age of the child. The IQ is calculated by dividing the mental age by the actual age, and multiplying by one hundred. In the case of a four year old who succeeds in the test at a level appropriate to a child of three years – we can say that he has a mental age of three years and an IQ of about seventy-five, which is at the lower end of the normal range of intelligence.

Parents may consider that this kind of measurement might be all right for *normal* children, but those with a handicapped child might well ask 'How can you expect my child to show his intelligence when he cannot use his hands, has no speech, and has had very little experience with these kinds of things?'

This is where the skill and expertise of the child psychologist comes in. It is his or her job to get through to the child's intelligence, and to search for the abilities, in spite of the presence of severe physical and speech handicaps. This can be done quite reliably with the majority of children. The experienced psychologist is more interested in assessing the handicapped child's *intentions*, rather than his actual performance in the tests. His attempts, however clumsy, to build a tower of graduated bricks, for example, are carefully observed and can provide quite convincing evidence that the child understands the problem of how things fit together in sequence; the fact that his tower of bricks may keep falling down is not important for this purpose. Most spastic children have enough motor control, however clumsy, to give a reliable indication of their intentions and of their understanding.

For those children more severely handicapped, some special tests and equipment are available, such as large scale bricks which interlock quite easily, and if even these are too difficult for the child physically, there are special tests that require practically no motor control or speech – the child merely has to point in the right direction, with his eyes or hands, in response to a series of questions, or simply to give some sign for 'yes' and 'no' in response to the questions, as the psychologist points to various objects and pictures. For example, given a series of pictures the psychologist can point to each one in turn, asking the child (after giving him training if necessary) to give some sort of sign when the picture is reached which represents, say, a bed, or 'the one we sleep in' or 'the one with four legs'.

On the whole, intelligence tests are not as reliable with handicapped children as they are with *normal* children, but in the hands of an experienced psychologist, who is knowledgeable about handicap and about the strengths and limitations of the tests, fairly useful results can be obtained.

Useful for what?

The chief purpose of the psychologist's tests of general intelligence is to provide *guide lines*. They tell us, at least approximately, how far a child has reached in his learning, and how much development in learning we may reasonably expect over the next few years. We have already pointed out the importance of an adult's 'expectations' about what a child should or should not be managing at certain stages in his life. If we expect too much, such as expecting a child of five years, whose mental age is around two years, to begin reading and do number work, disappointment is bound to ensue. Both the child and his parents are likely to become extremely frustrated. Alternatively, if we expect too little we may miss the chance of improving our child's learning, at a stage when he is receptive and ready to learn.

Numerous studies have shown that just over 50% of children with cerebral palsy are of more or less normal intelligence. Just under 25% are slow learning children (with mental ages between about half and three-quarters of normal: IQ 50-75), and the remaining 25% are very slow learning (mental ages rather below a normal child of half their age, IQ below 50). These children whose intelligence is subnormal usually have more severe physical handicaps, both being the result of extensive impairment to the brain cells, but this is not always the case and there are a few startling exceptions. A small number of extremely handicapped children have a high intelligence, whilst some quite mildly handicapped children are markedly subnormal. Since nearly half of the cerebral palsied children are retarded in their intelligence (compared to about 2% amongst the *normal*, non-cerebral palsied population) it is essential that we should modify our expectations about their rate of learning and our methods of teaching.

How Can Parents Help in Stimulating Their Handicapped Child?

Some people might question the point of trying to improve the performance of a severely handicapped child. They might argue that his skills are so limited that the time and effort are scarcely worthwhile. Any parent after a tiring day will expect to feel the same on many occasions!

However, anyone who has observed a child in a handicapped children's play group, struggling with determination and persistence to master some task that they have observed other children performing, and has seen the delight which accompanies success, will realise that achievement is as important to the handicapped, as it is to any child. Indeed, one might argue that the smallest steps towards self-help in dressing, feeding and moving around take on a greater significance in the life of the handicapped child, whose horizons are necessarily so limited. The parents' aim should be to encourage the child's efforts in self-help skills, ensuring that any task is almost within the child's reach, so that continued disappointment does not dampen his eagerness.

A good example would be in the business of dressing, do not suddenly decide 'the child should try to put on his shoes today' and leave him to it. Do the first part of the action for him, putting the shoe on his toe and helping him to pull it over his heel. After success in this, the parent may each time leave a little more of the action to be managed by the child so that eventually he finishes up by doing the whole thing himself. If there is no improvement in skill after several attempts, *leave it*, realising that your sights have been set too high and try something simpler. Teaching a new skill is a subtle compromise between you doing too much that he could manage himself, and setting so hard a task that failure is bound to ensue, or it takes so long that the child's concentration is lost.

We can summarise the most effective ways of encouraging learning, as follows:-

INTERESTING TASKS – Some severely handicapped children do not, in the early years, seem to show much curiosity, or eagerness to learn. The parent must therefore work towards stimulating his interest, by using large bright toys and materials, including something different each week that he has not seen before, or has not seen for a long time, so that an element of novelty is kept up.

SHORT SESSIONS – Set aside one or two periods of say twenty minutes each day, for carrying out some fairly concentrated learning. This is better than trying to carry on for hours at a time – children concentrate

206

and achieve quite a lot in fairly short spurts, with rest and relaxation in between.

SET A TARGET – It helps both parents and the child to aim at a goal; it enables us to be aware of progress, and to get satisfaction from knowing when we reach a certain goal, or nearly do so. These goals can be very simple, depending on the mental age of the child, ranging from very simple activities in building with bricks, or putting objects in and out of containers, to matching shapes or colour cards or jigsaws for a slow learning five year old and so on.

SMALL STEPS – Choose simple activities and break them down into manageable steps. For example, with a game like 'Picture Lotto', the matching of pictures can start with a few obviously different pictures, moving gradually to matching those in which the differences between the pictures are more subtle. Give plenty of practice and opportunities for repetition.

ENCOURAGEMENT– Give plenty of praise for success – praising for effort, as well as for actual accomplishment; play down failure as much as possible, without showing surprise or irritation.

If these general principles are kept in mind, the mastering of the simplest skill will bring with it much satisfaction to the child. Learning can be enjoyable!

Special Learning Difficulties

Some handicapped children with normal intelligence and relatively minor physical handicap may nevertheless have very unevenly developed learning abilities. For example, they may be very good with words, conversing readily, using sentences well at an early age, but be extremely poor at practical things, such as handling constructional toys or dressing. These are children with special learning difficulties and the unevenness in their mental development calls for careful psychological assessment and advice. We still have a great deal to learn about such children.

One important group are those with perceptual handicaps.

Perceptual Handicaps

Visual perception is the ability to recognise and distinguish between shapes, such as a circle and a square, to distinguish between the outline of a drawing and its surrounding background and to recognise different directions in space, (left and right, up and down, etc.) especially in relation to one's own body. Such children are easily confused about which direction to take, and how to get their bodies past obstacles, their arms into sleeves and so on.

They may also have difficulty in relating what they see, to what they hear and to what they touch. In other words their different senses do not hang together very well. For example, the *normal* baby at six months of age not only hears a sound, but will usually turn his head and look enquiringly round attempting to identify what might be making the sound. His hearing, vision, motor control and intelligence have, over the months, worked together to accomplish this; whereas the child having perceptual handicaps (although the separate senses of hearing, vision and touch etc., might be all right in themselves) cannot link these up, or rather, may be extremely slow in learning to do so.

This linking-up of visual and motor performance is very important, since we use our visual perception a good deal in ordinary life – indeed a great part of the information we receive from our surroundings comes from the eyes, and is then interpreted by the brain. We then usually act on the information we have gained and make some sort of motor or vocal response. In short, we integrate vision with movement. The *normal* baby starts to do this during the first months of life, e.g. he watches his own hand movements, or reaches for a toy. One can thus begin to imagine the confusions of a child with visual perceptual handicaps, who might have normal abilities in other directions.

In helping the child with perceptual handicaps, we have, as is often the case with handicapped children, to encourage and teach things that come more or less automatically to the ordinary child. Otherwise they may tend to shy away from what they find difficult – visual judgment in this case, and over develop (sometimes rather superficially) what might come more easily, such as speech and appreciation of language. In short they become great talkers and poor doers.

Therefore, lots of encouragement and opportunities are needed to help bring on a child's appreciation of shape and patterns and to link up these perceptions with the use of his hands. There is plenty of material available for this, described in the chapter on play, such as simple formboards, posting boxes, graduated beakers, boxes of bricks. For slightly older children, of mental age three and over, there are sets of colour and shape-sorting games which can be helpful, and games involving paper and pencil, such as copying very simple lines and shapes, and finishing incomplete drawings.

If a child is good with words, use them to help his visual judgment, e.g. naming a circle, pointing out its similarity to a football, and so help him distinguish between that and an oval or egg-shape one. One formboard inset can be described as like a roof another like a tunnel.

Some handicapped children show a short attention span and are easily distracted from the task in hand by an extraneous sound, such as a lorry passing, or the sight of a curtain swaying in the wind. With children who are so easily diverted, a helpful move is to cut down the amount of distraction around them; therefore, for our teaching and training periods we should use a quiet corner of the room and keep it fairly plain and bare, tidying other toys out of sight and presenting the child with only a few pieces of equipment at a time. This helps him to focus his attention and eventually to get more satisfaction from what he is doing (one learns very little if one is flitting from one thing to another) so that eventually, as he becomes older, he can cope with ordinary surroundings. Most psychologists regard these perceptual and attention handicaps as a kind of time-lag in the child's development, rather than a permanent impairment, i.e. the attention and perception of the handicapped child is often at a level appropriate to a much younger child; the techniques we have briefly described may help to speed up the maturation of the child.

Motor And Speech Expression – The Output From The Child

We have been considering various factors to do with the way a child learns – the input of impressions through his various senses, and the intelligence, perception and attention that enable him to organise and make sense of these impressions, and we will now mention the 'output' as it were, from the child; his means of expression through speech, hand control, gesture, etc.

The psychologist is very interested in children whose communication difficulties are such that they cannot properly express their intelligence – either through speech or hand movements. We have already mentioned some of the ways in which the psychologist communicates with severely handicapped children, such as by providing toys and test situations in which the adult can do the talking and movements, and the child merely has to signal 'yes' or 'no' at the right time. Parents can practise this sort of communication with their very handicapped child. For example, the child of mental age three, without speech or much hand control can get stimulation and enjoyment from a simple picture – say of a street scene, which the parent can talk about – and then ask questions – 'is this the policeman?' – 'is this the ice cream van?' pointing to various parts of the picture in turn and waiting for the child to give some sign for 'yes' when the correct part is reached.

For older children without speech, but having reasonable hand and arm control, a simple system of gesture may be useful – such as the 'Hundred Gestures' developed by L.M. Levett at Meldreth Manor School, which enables a completely speechless child to communicate simple ideas and needs – such as for food, drink and toileting.

For less handicapped children, the range of aids described by Nancie Finnie – (for example, play material that does not slip around the table too much) is of great help in reducing the frustrations that beset a child who may have lots of ideas, but no easy means of expressing them. For older children, of mental age five plus, a great variety of aids are available to assist in reading, writing and number work – aids that take the drudgery out of writing, such as rubber stamps for letters and numbers, and typewriters; all of which are particularly useful for school work.

Stimulating Environments

We have discussed the various factors within the child that influence his learning – his drive to learn and the basic physical and mental equipment that enables him to do so. Very little of this learning would actually take place without the stimulation offered by the parents and we have talked about some of the ways in which this stimulation can be stepped up and improved – by gaining a deeper understanding of how children learn, getting our expectations and goals right, setting realistic targets and trying out various ways of reaching these targets, and so on. The psychologist can help parents, particularly in respect of their child's intellectual and educational development; and, in collaboration with those other experts represented in this book, the whole team (including the parents) can work towards the fullest possible understanding of the child's strengths and weaknesses and plan for the best possible treatment, training and education.

In this chapter we have tended to concentrate our efforts on the child who is more severely physically handicapped and slow learning, and for whom the setting of realistic goals is very important if frustration is to be avoided; the blending of a realistic approach, with reasonable optimism is not easy to achieve by the parents of these very handicapped children. It takes years.

Throughout those years, we must remember Professor Jack Tizard's comment – that childhood is not only a preparation for later life and adulthood; it is life. Childhood is to be enjoyed by both child and the parents, without continually having one eye on the child's future; he lives for the present also. In other words, we must avoid overdoing our training and teaching. Certainly the handicapped child needs some extra stimulation to make up for what he would otherwise miss; there should be short periods in the day of intense stimulation, together with time for rest, relaxation and letting off steam.

Chapter 16

THE FUNDAMENTALS OF GRASP AND MANIPULATION

Independence in any activity is only possible when the child has symmetry, head control, eye-hand co-ordination, the ability to grasp and to release regardless of the position of his arms, movement at his hips enabling him to reach out in any direction, sufficient sitting balance to sit without having to rely on his hands. Before considering the link between play and everyday activities it is necessary to understand the developmental sequences that lead to the use of the hands for future skills.

Turn to Appendix 1, and read 'Early Stages of Normal Development', and you will see how the development of the hands evolves at the same time as the gross motor patterns of movement which underlie all skills; for example, until the child can use his hands for support grasp and release he will be unable to get off the floor independently or in fact be independent in any activity. The child learns and practises many of these movements while he is being handled by his mother and later while he plays.

In the sequences of *normal* development, the 'reaching' of the eyes precedes the 'reaching' of the arms and hands, both appearing long before manipulation begins.

The first object that holds the baby's gaze is the face of his mother. It is not merely a fleeting glance, but an *intense* gaze while she nurses, plays and handles him, especially when he takes his bottle. At this time he also starts to be aware of the human voice, particularly that of his mother – smiling when he sees her face and when he hears her speak.

With the cerebral palsied child we are sometimes inclined to neglect this opportunity for communication between mother and child, possibly understandably so, as handling generally takes a long time and admittedly controlling the child may be difficult, nevertheless as a very important phase of development it must form part of any programme for early handling.

Experiment so as to find the best position, a symmetrical one which will enable you to be *face to face* with your baby, begin at a distance say of about 6″. For the more severely handicapped child you may have to start with him in side-lying, progressing later to a more practicable position. Good control of the head and shoulders of the child is essential when you are speaking and trying to get his attention. Give him plenty of opportunities to appreciate the variety of tones in your voice, sometimes even singing to him. It is important to remember to do this not only when he is lying flat on his back, but also when he is being lifted and nursed. Getting his attention in this way will help him not only to focus on your face, but to pay attention to your voice and to his own sounds with their varying pitch and tone.

Symmetry, as we have said, enables the *normal* baby to bring his arms forward and to get his hands together; his arms at this stage will be abducted at the shoulders. This enables him not only to touch, clasp and unclasp his fingers, but also to look at them, he does this many times a day and for many weeks, soon being able to maintain the grasp of the hands while he rolls from his back to his side.

When helping the cerebral palsied child to clasp and unclasp his hands it is important to see that he does not press his arms against his chest, as this will result in the firm closure of his hands and making eye contact with them impossible. Do *not* be satisfied with merely helping him to bring his arms forward with closed hands, but see that the hands are open before coming into contact with each other, for only in this way will he have a chance to feel the palms of his hands and to touch and move his own hands and fingers. See if he can grasp his hands while, for example, you roll him from side to side; if grasping should make his elbows very bent, get him to hold his hands together with straight arms.

The *normal* baby then starts to learn more about his hands and fingers by taking them to his mouth to suck and feel them with his lips and tongue, later he will start to explore his lips, cheeks and tongue with his fingers.

This early exploration of the mouth may be very difficult for the cerebral palsied child, as the added stimulus of putting his fingers inside his mouth may be so strong that it will result in increased extensor spasticity, the child's head, shoulders and arms and even his body pushing backwards. For such children, oral therapy will be the first step and your speech therapist will show you how to do this.

It is important that you find a position in which the cerebral palsied child can not only bring his own hands together, but at the same time, can see them and take them to his mouth. Assess your child's difficulties and then decide whether, on his tummy, side-lying, using a wedge or baby rocker is most suitable; when you are helping him you may find that a position on your lap is the best. While you handle him throughout the day encourage him to become familiar with his hands, for example, when giving him his bottle place his open hands around it. As in any new activity it is only by constant repetition that the child learns, give him every opportunity to support himself on his hands, to grasp and release.

The sketches at the end of this chapter depict ways to help you when the child progresses to the stage of self-exploration, and later, when he starts to reach out to touch the faces of those playing with him.

Co-ordination between hands and eyes starts when the *normal* baby sees an object that he wants and makes a purposeful movement to reach towards it, he waves his arms about and he does so first with *both* arms; it is interesting to note that at the same time as he does this he opens and closes his hands in anticipation of grasping the object, which at this stage he is unable to do. This is not merely the beginning of eye-hand co-ordination but is teaching the baby something about the distance between himself and an object, i.e. how far he has to reach out to touch it. He then progresses to reaching out for, and touching the object, finally having the ability to reach, touch, grasp and manipulate.

The athetoid child has little difficulty in attempting to reach out, but because of his fluctuating postural tone and involuntary movements he lacks fixation, as a result all his movements are disorganised being poorly timed and directed. He will reach out with one arm which, in his case, will probably go out to the side before coming forward, making eye-hand control, and eventually grasping, very difficult.

The spastic child, owing to his spasticity, will be restricted in his ability to reach out, any excitement will most likely result in making him stiffer, his arms bending and being pressed against his body, alternatively he may reach out but with stiffly extended arms, which are turned in at the shoulders, with a fisted hand.

Refer again to 'Early Stages of Normal Development' and to the sections dealing with vision and eye-hand co-ordination which lead to the *normal* child having the ability first to reach out and grasp – a very gradual process.

It is obviously a waste of time to expect, or to try to encourage, a child with cerebral palsy to learn to reach out and play if we first do nothing about his *basic* problems. Start by *encouraging* your child to reach out when you go to pick him up and get him to hold his own arm up and forward when you wash or dress him, lead him gradually to co-operate in these activities encouraging him to grasp when he loses his balance and so forth.

Tactile experiences are important for all young children, but particularly so for the cerebral palsied child who either has a fisted hand, or one that opens and closes when touching a surface. *Do not* have special sessions for giving the child different sensory experiences, using, for example, small squares or pieces of material, these experiences should be gained throughout the day with such everyday objects as your clothes, the various materials of chairs, curtains, carpets, rough and smooth towels and other objects inside and outside the house – in fact sensory experiences of all things that surround him and that he comes into contact with during the day.

For more advanced skills the child will need the ability to grasp regardless of the position of his arm and to dissociate the movement of the fingers one from the other, for example to point with the index finger, to flex fingers independently from one to another and to apply this ability to function.

It should be noted that at the same time as the child starts to become

213

more proficient in the use of his hands, speech starts to develop which often helps him with the task in hand; at about this time we start to show the child his first picture books, encouraging him to point out the objects we describe, to turn over the pages and eventually to name them.

Due to his total abnormal patterns the cerebral palsied child often has problems of combining manipulation and speech. It is therefore important that we encourage him to speak as he uses his hands, not only to give him an understanding of language, so important for future speech, *but also to help him to start organising his thoughts so as to reinforce his actions.* Many of the points brought out in the foregoing are illustrated in figs. 164 to 184.

Finally when thinking of the ways in which you can help your child to use his hands do not think merely of them in relation to toys, remember that to learn to grasp and manipulate is basic to all activities and the only way to ensure independence.

As the child gets older and starts to co-operate with his washing, dressing, feeding and so on, whilst we may encourage him to become independent and to use his hands, we so often *fail to give him the practice he needs* in the early stages which he can so easily have *throughout all his waking hours* and which forms a valuable link between handling and treatment.

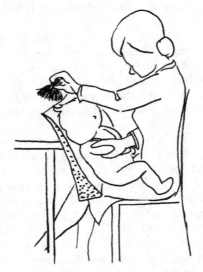

Figure 164. The child sits astride his mother's lap facing her, she prevents movement between his head and arms by holding his arms in front of his chest. He is encouraged to look at and follow the woolly ball – which has a small bell attached – as she moves it from mid-line to the side. On other occasions she will hold his head still, getting him to follow the ball in different directions with his eyes only. The child's ability to focus and possible line of vision at various stages in his development *must always* be taken into account.

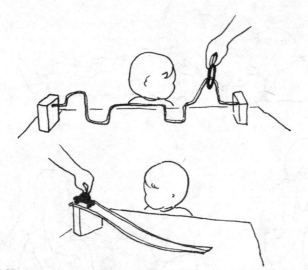

Figure 165. As the child sits at a table he is encouraged to follow the object at first with *his eyes only.* In the sketch the movement of the object is from left to right then right to left, up and down, towards and away from him and diagonally across should be included later. Progress would be for the child to do a similar movement tracing with his index finger, dipped first in finger-paint, across the table while he follows the movement of his finger, finally doing the same movement with an object in his hands.

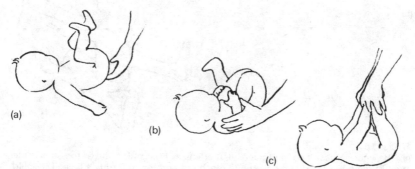

(a)

(b)

(c)

Figure 166

(a) If the child is to be encouraged to look at and at the same time to hold his feet, see that not only the hips but the lower part of his spine are off the support. Many children when they try to reach out for their toes push their head back and this immediately straightens their hips and legs.

(b) When the child takes his toes to his mouth see that the legs are bent and turned out, help by keeping his arms forward and up at the shoulder. With the effort of taking his foot to his mouth the bending of one leg may make the other leg straighten and the child will often lose his balance. To prevent this happening have your other hand under the opposite hip. Work as quickly as possible to get him to hold both feet at once, taking one or both to his mouth.

(c) A child normally plays for many hours in this position, i.e. holding his toes while the legs remain straight and moving his legs up and down. Work for this pattern which is a good preparation for long-sitting later on, but do see that the legs are not stiff or turned in.

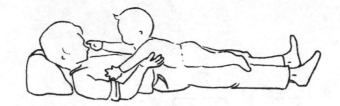

(a)

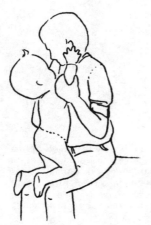

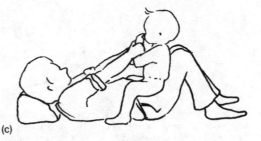

(c)

(b)

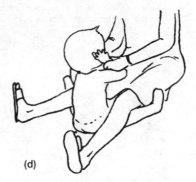

(d)

Figure 167

(a) The young *spastic* child in the sketch practises lifting his head at the same time straightening his back, as he learns to reach out and touch Daddy's face. The child is held under his chest, the shoulders are kept up and forward and weight is taken by the child on one arm while he reaches out with the other.

(b) A more advanced position with bent knees and straight hips, there will be a greater tendency for the arms to press down and bend in this position.

(c) The child sits astride you, his feet flat on the floor. He takes your hands to touch his face, ears, shoulders and so on – at intervals give support with your knees. When he starts to take his own hands to his face, control him under the top of his arms turning them out at the shoulders and stopping them from pressing down.

(d) A good position for the *spastic* child who finds it difficult to sit with his hips bent, legs straight apart and turned out. Controlling his legs with yours in this way leaves your hands free to *help him*. In this instance both his hands are placed on his ears with *open* hands he should progress to holding onto his ear lobes with finger and thumb, the palm facing towards his face. If his elbows start to pull in, change your grip and support him under the upper arm, keep his elbows out.

216

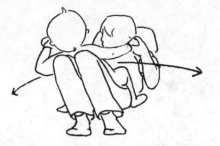

Figure 168. A *spastic* child with poor head and trunk control sits astride his father who gives support to the child's back with his legs. The father moves his legs sideways teaching the child to make the necessary adjustment of his head and trunk as he learns to balance in preparation for sitting without support and to be able to use his hands. The child is encouraged to grasp his father's hands, keeping his arms straight out in front *of him.* If the child's arms feel heavy and push down, take his arms above his head, keeping them straight and turned out at the shoulder.

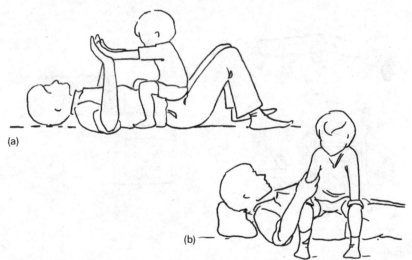

(a)

(b)

Figure 169
These two sketches show the *athetoid* child. An appreciation of body awareness is as important to the *athetoid* as to the *spastic,* but the *techniques of control differ.* The *athetoid* moves too much, and we have to give him a feeling of stability. This can be done through the head, shoulders or hips.
(a) The child grasps your hands while you pull him towards you keeping his arms straight, then quickly jerk him back a little. This will give him the feeling of grasping while at the same time you increase the tone in his trunk (making it firm) and improve his head control. Try also to encourage him to push against your hands, this will give him the very important pattern of reaching forward in a controlled way.
(b) The child is controlled firmly at the shoulder, the arm is turned in and kept straight by his side. He puts his hands on his knees and moves slowly forward to put his hands on his feet, in front of his feet and beside his feet, returning to the sitting position with his hands on his knees. Take your hands away as soon as possible.

217

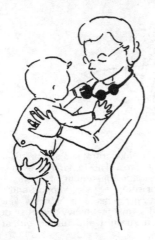
(a)

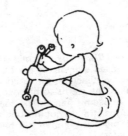
(b)

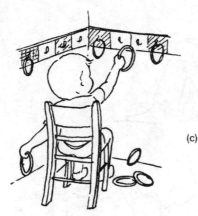
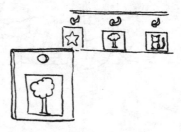
(c)

Figure 170
These captions illustrate various stages of grasping.
(a) Grandmother has a string of large wooden red balls around her neck, the child
sits astride her hip in such a way that enables him to bring both hands forward,
being face to face she can speak to him as he plays. Little bells, hoops, squares
of foam can also be used, start by using one only and gradually increase the
number on the string.
(b) The child has acquired sitting balance but feels insecure when attempting to
use both hands. An inflated rubber ring, as illustrated, or a similar shape in foam
will provide the extra confidence he needs. The child is grasping dowel rods with
bells attached. Rods with flags, windmills or sleeves of different colours or textures
over the rods can be used.
(c) The older child practises his ability to grasp by hanging up different coloured
rings. He can also use matching squares, or matching plywood squares with
pictures which he places on the appropriate square on the hook, this requires a
finer type of grasp. In this way the child combines movement of the whole body
with eye-hand control and the ability to grasp and release as the arm is moved in
different directions.

218

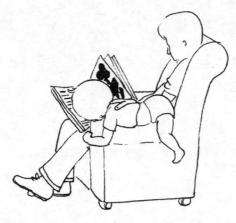

Figure 171. The child lies over the arm of the chair (see note) feeling its texture and comparing it with the textures in the pictures in the book, which is made specifically for that purpose. For the older child upright-kneeling, standing, facing the back of the chair or sitting in the chair, then moving to one of these other positions should be tried.

Note: If the child is very asymmetrical this will mean, for example, that if his tone is high *(spasticity)* that this increase in tone will often affect the cheeks, tongue and so on; be careful if he lies as illustrated that you do *not* have his more affected side against the support.

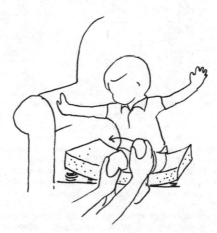

Figure 172. If the child is to use his hands for later skills, good balance is essential. By placing a square of foam on the base of a chair, as illustrated, balance reactions can be facilitated, this can also be done with the child astride a roller.

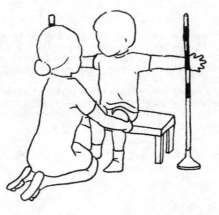

Figure 173. Playing with two sticks, as illustrated, is a simple way of teaching the child to grasp regardless of the position of his head, a difficulty that often arises when he starts to dress and undress himself. Start with his arms out at the sides, straight and turned out at the shoulders, this will help him keep his back straight. He should gradually learn to do the following movements with the sticks at first out at his sides, as illustrated, and then in front of him, keeping his head in the middle and looking at you – as in (1) and (2) below. In (3) and (4) however he looks at his hands as he grasps and lets go of the sticks.

(1) Grasp both sticks, arms remaining straight and steady.

(2) Letting go a stick with one hand and grasping again, without any movement in the other arm.

(3) Turning his head to look at his hand, as he grasps and lets go of one stick. He may need help in keeping the other arm straight while he does this.

(4) Grasping and letting go of one stick with his head turned away from it. To make this more amusing, stick strips of coloured tape on the sticks and ask the child to grasp a particular colour, or for the older child numbers. The mother in the illustration holds the child's legs together; as one of the most common difficulties found in the cerebral palsied child is the inability to perform independent movements of the head, arms and hands, the legs often part or the pelvis turns upsetting the child's balance.

(5) The two sticks should eventually be placed in front of the child.

220

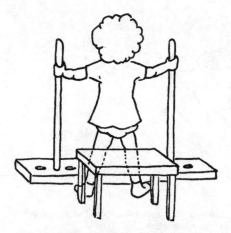

Figure 174. A way of combining grasp with movement; the poles are placed in the holes at the extremities of the board, this calls for the widest extension of the child's arms, eventually the two poles are placed in the holes directly in front of him. The child is encouraged to get up from sitting and vice-versa. The variety of hand movements suggested in figure 173 can also be used; to begin with, the plank (with holes) is used to provide stability and it can gradually be discarded as the child reaches the stage of being able to walk with sticks.

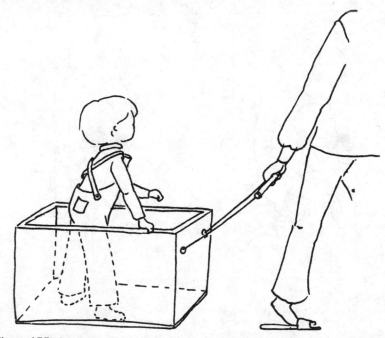

Figure 175. An enjoyable way of learning to balance while developing automatically arm-support and grasp, later the child can learn to push and pull the box himself.

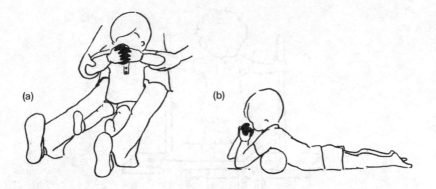

(a)

(b)

Figure 176. Two positions that can be used to encourage the child to hold and bring an orange towards his mouth.
(a) Sitting between your legs, the child's head and shoulders can be kept forward and your legs help to keep the arms away from his body. Support under the elbows enables the child to lift the orange to his mouth.
(b) The child lies over a roller which keeps his arms forward at the shoulder and brings the orange to his mouth instead of vice versa. He may need help to keep his hips down.

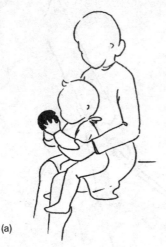

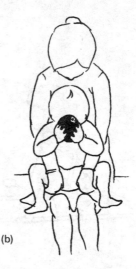

(a)

(b)

Figure 177
(a) The child sits astride your leg to keep his legs apart and hips bent. You help him lift his arms by supporting under the elbows and pulling them away from his body as he takes the orange to his mouth.
(b) Where the arms are fairly good but moving them, immediately makes the hips straighten and the legs go very stiff and turn in, control him at the thighs turning the legs out and keeping the hips bent, as illustrated.

222

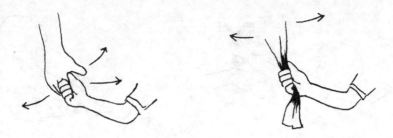

Figure 178. By grasping your fingers and later by holding a towel in his hand, the child's arm can be moved in all directions while he tries to retain his grasp. This can be followed by the child moving your arm in all directions while you hold the towel. The child should only practise the movements in a position in which he has good balance and does not need an arm to support himself.

Note: Your finger and the towel are placed across the palm and then out between the thumb and index finger.

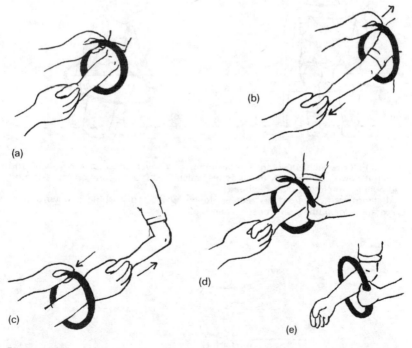

Figure 179
(a) Grasp the child's hand and the ring.
(b) Pull the child's arm through the ring taking the ring up to his shoulder while he says 'push'.
(c) Pushing the child's arm out of the ring while he says 'pull'.
(d) The child holds the ring and your hand, and he pulls and pushes with your help.
(e) Finally he holds the ring on his own and repeats the same movements.

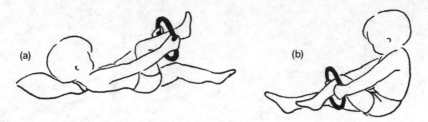

Figure 180
(a) The same sequence of movements, the child lying on his back. Here he pulls and pushes the ring over his leg.
(b) The same sequence of movements. but done in sitting on the floor.

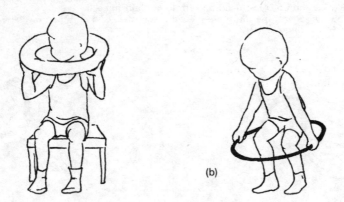

Figure 181
(a) Sitting on a stool pushing a 'swimming ring' over and above his head and pulling it down again, finally as far as his waist. This is a preparation for taking off and pulling on clothes over his head.
(b) Pulling the hoop from his feet up to his waist and pushing it down again; preparation for putting on trousers, pants etc.

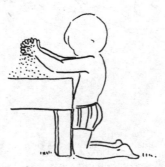

Figure 182. Playing with sand helps to teach the child the movements necessary for washing his hands.

224

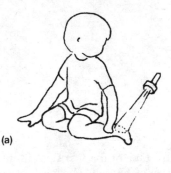

(a)

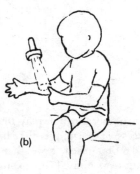

(b)

Figure 183. Shine the torch on the child's leg and then get him to look and touch. Move the light about quite quickly so that he moves and looks for the light at the same time.
(a) and (b) he rubs the spot of light with his hand, later he rubs the spot of light holding a flannel or sponge.

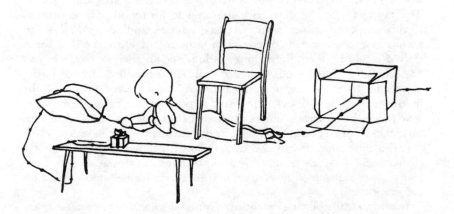

Figure 184. An 'obstacle course' made by leading a piece of rope under and over various objects teaches a child more about himself in relation to objects and to use his hands for support and grasp as he makes his way to the end of the rope. As an incentive for effort drop a small 'prize' in a box attached to the end of the rope so that he has to unwrap the parcel to get his prize.

Chapter 17

PLAY

It is mainly through play that a child learns. One of the first steps in this process of learning is that he becomes aware of himself. Having become aware of himself, he is then ready to explore and learn about others in relation to himself, for example, to touch and point to his mother's face, eyes and mouth. In time when we ask him 'where is my nose?' 'where is your mouth?' he will point and touch; he then goes a step further and learns the names of the parts which he touches. Later he can explain, 'my mouth is under my nose', 'my ears are at the side of my head'.

As his field of recognition widens, he uses and relates what he has learned to his dolls and toys. Later, as he crawls and moves about he becomes aware of himself in space and discovers that there are two sides to his body; that his head is at the top and his feet at the bottom; that his chest and tummy are in front, and his back and bottom are at the back. He later makes use of such information as he starts to feed, wash and dress himself.

A child also has to learn and to understand how the world around him works. He learns as he plays to differentiate between shapes and textures. This he does when he starts to take things to his mouth. He learns also to differentiate between sizes, weights, colours and so forth; how to manipulate objects and to assess the amount of effort needed for a desired result. He learns how things fit into one another, or how they can be screwed or unscrewed, squeezed, pushed, or pulled. By exploring objects he learns to understand where are the top, bottom, sides, the inside and outside of objects. He learns to perceive and calculate distance; how far he has to reach out before he can get hold of and pick up his toys; the width and height of things and their relationship to one another.

In learning what he can and cannot do with things around him – his environment – he learns to rattle toys, to bang, to throw, to build. He also realises that some things are good to taste and smell and that others are unpleasant.

Learning while playing extends to climbing in and out, up and down, under, over and around objects, finding out the space through which he can squeeze, what heights are dangerous to jump from and what can be safely managed. All this, and more besides, the child learns while he plays, becoming more skilful as he grows older, doing more and more for himself, asking questions and practising and learning from his mistakes.

The Normal Baby

If you watch a *normal* baby while he plays, one thing will immediately strike you – he is never still and he is seldom silent, though to begin with he just gurgles and babbles as he plays. A baby lying on his back and playing with his toys continually kicks his legs and wriggles about. When he is able to lie on his tummy, he is just as active. Interspersed with his play, he rocks on his tummy, lifting and waving his arms about as he kicks his legs. He pivots on his tummy, rolls over on his back still clutching his toys and taking them to his mouth. As he acquires balance and control in sitting, in upright kneeling and in crawling, he moves continually from one position to another as he plays with his toys.

In this way, besides practising new patterns of movement, the baby learns about himself in space and about his relationship to things around him. Later he tries to grasp a toy that is out of reach and realises that he must move towards it. A ball rolls under a chair and he has to work out how to get it. He climbs on to a chair to get a toy and has to decide which is the best way of getting down without dropping it. He bumps his pushcart into the furniture until he realises that the furniture is solid and he must find his way around it. He discovers that some things go faster if pushed, others if pulled.

The Cerebral Palsied Child

Play is equally important for the cerebral palsied child. He, too, must become aware of himself, explore and get to know his hands, face, feet and so forth; learn about himself in relation to others, and understand how the world around him works. Because of his difficulties, in moving and balancing, in eye-hand co-ordination – and often with the additional handicap of defects in seeing and hearing – he needs a lot of help. Owing to his difficulty in listening, in looking at what he is doing, in touching, holding and manipulating objects, his progress will be slow and he will need considerable understanding and guidance. His span of concentration and his ability to remember are often of short duration. His handicap prevents him from learning through play in a natural way, so, unless he has help and encouragement, he will not be able to learn as he plays or to reach his potential.

The Severely Handicapped or Very Young Cerebral Palsied Child

How can we help the severely handicapped child, who is restricted in his movements and has no sitting balance, to use his hands for play? We should first try to analyse his difficulties and find positions which will enable him to use his hands to the best advantage, that will be easiest for eye-hand co-ordination and will present the least difficulties for balance. He is at his best when lying on his side – or on his tummy. Lying flat on the floor is not satisfactory. Even a normal person soon finds this position uncomfortable, and especially tiring if at the same time trying to do something with his hands. The sketches in chapter 13 show how with

227

the use of a roller, bolster or prone board, the child can adapt himself to lying on his tummy, making it possible for him to keep his head up and his back straight, to bring his arms forward, and to start to use his hands.

Some points to remember when deciding on a good position for play:
The child should not remain in any one position for more than twenty minutes.
A variety of positions should be tried before deciding which is the best. It is not necessary to keep to the same position each day, for his problems, although basically the same, will vary to some degree. What was good yesterday may not be so good today. For example, some days when lying on his tummy he may keep turning his head too far to the side and roll onto his back. For this you may need to give him extra support at the side of his chest, or make some adaptations that will keep his shoulders and arms forward. It is important that you notice these changes or the child who is unable to use his hands may become frustrated and cease to make any effort to use them.
Although a baby *normally* first plays when lying on his back, this is usually the worst position for the cerebral palsied child. Some children cannot get their shoulders and arms forward and are therefore unable to put their hands together. Others may be able to get their arms forward only to hold them tightly over the chest, bent at the elbows and with hands clenched which they are unable to open to reach out for a toy. Figs. 137 and 140, pages 180/1 show how these problems can be overcome, to some extent, by having the baby in a 'Bouncing Cradle', or for the older child a hammock.
Many children who are so handicapped when on their backs are also unable to lift their heads when lying on their tummies, even when well supported. Figs. 185 a) b), shows how, by having the child on your lap you can get him accustomed to lying on his tummy while you control his head and keep his shoulders and arms forward. Immediately you feel that he is trying to control his head himself, be sure to take your hands gently away. Some children find it easier to lie with their arms straight; others with them bent taking weight on their elbows. Try both ways, as the child will eventually have to manage with his arms forward in all positions and to take weight on them.
When the child has achieved some sitting balance the chairs and tables described in chapter 12 can be tried and adapted.

First Steps In Helping the Child to Play
During the first two years an important part of play is by imitation both of sounds and movements – saying 'bye-bye', clapping hands, playing 'pat-a-cake', looking into a mirror, breathing onto and touching it with his fingers, playing 'peep-bo', and so on. Help the child with the various gestures, repeating the simple phrases for him, and be sure that he can

both see what he is doing and hear what you are saying. Later use such rhymes as, 'This is the way we wash our hands', and 'Simon says do this, Simon says do that', which teach him not only to move, but also to learn the names of parts of his body. Use phrases that describe everyday activities, and encourage him to repeat the rhymes with you. His span of concentration will be very short at first so repeat a few actions and phrases for short periods until he really becomes familiar with them.

At this stage the child will discover that he can make new sounds. Encourage him to repeat them by copying him. A good way of making this into a game is by joining together two hollow cardboard cylinders with a piece of string, making them into a telephone. If you cover one end with wax paper, you will find that the sounds will be magnified.

Helping Him to Use His Hands

If you look again at the sketches in chapter 4, you will notice how the abnormal postures of the cerebral palsied child make it impossible for him to bring his arms forward with hands together, or to bring his hands towards his body with the palms facing him. In some cases the hands are permanently closed, or else they close only when the head is turned away from the arm, thereby making it impossible for him to look at his hand. In other cases the hands are permanently open, or else open directly the arm is lifted.

To use our hands adequately we must be able to hold our head steady. This enables us to look at what we are doing and to open our hands to grasp and release regardless of the position of the arms. It is a waste of time to place a toy into the hand of a child who has no head control and who is unable to release, and expect him to play with it.

A *normal* baby spends many hours just looking at his hands, moving them in front of his face, bringing them together and feeling them, putting them to his mouth and so on, before he learns to use them purposefully; the length of time he continues to do this is an indication of the importance this kind of hand play has in his development.

A first step with the cerebral palsied child, is to help him to become aware of his hands, making it possible for him to feel, grasp and release, before giving him actual objects to handle. When the baby reaches the stage of being able to bring his hands into mid-line, at this time often clutching and grasping his vest, try placing a piece of thin foam, tissue, newspaper, tin-foil or other material over his chest tucking it in around his sides, this is a good way to encourage tactile sensation.

The importance of a good position of head, trunk control and, particularly, of good control at the shoulders to enable him to use his hands, has been described in earlier chapters. Helping the child to learn about his own face and body, an important link for future play is described in chapter 16.

In addition to the suggestions made in chapter 16, the following ideas can be tried to help the child become 'aware' of his hands.

Shine a torch, preferably one with different colours, over his hands and through his fingers. Draw his attention to the various patterns and shadows his hands and fingers make on a wall or table.

Wind a piece of rough string or bright ribbon through his fingers, leaving two long loose ends to encourage him to pull it.

Use different coloured thimbles to attract his attention to his fingers, getting him to bang and to scratch a flat surface.

Draw a face on the palm and the backs of his hands.

When he is able to use his hands a little, encourage him to put his hand in a jar filled with rice, lentils, beans, macaroni, lump sugar, and let him move it around as he wishes, encouraging him to take the contents in and out of the jar.

The same objects can be placed on a tray and you can get him to sweep them to the top, bottom or sides of the tray. Be sure to make him aware, as you play with him, that his hands are moving from side to side, up and down, or in the middle of the tray; if possible get him to repeat or say with you the direction in which he is moving his hands.

Encourage him to explore inside a paper bag full of well-defined objects that are known to him and then let him play as he wishes. In many cases just to feel and move the things around is achievement and a process of learning.

Slowly and repeatedly rub his hands, including his fingers, over different surfaces, using everyday objects such as fruit, bread, household objects and so on, till he feels the whole object in his hands and becomes aware of the texture, contour and edges. Always name the objects, their shape, colour and the way they feel as he handles them. He must become aware of the object as a whole before he can appreciate the individual parts and their relationship to one another. This is often very difficult for the cerebral palsied child.

Place his fingers into salt, sugar, jam, or around a bowl that has held cream, custard or a mixture that he likes. The severely handicapped child can only enjoy these experiences of feeling, smelling and tasting if objects are brought and introduced to him. For example, if it should be snowing, even bring in a bucket of snow for him to handle.

Playing and learning here are synonymous. Give him as wide a range of experience as you can, including the stimulation of feeling, smelling, seeing and listening, and encourage him all the time to express himself by gesture and, whenever possible, of course, by speech.

Playing with your child should not be a special half-hour session a day but should be included in the daily routine. Make use of the things around you; when in the bedroom let him look at himself in the mirror, feel the difference between the blankets and the sheets and help you pull them into position, the difference between the soft pillows and the hard mattress, let him bounce on the mattress, in the bathroom let him try the taps, feel the difference between a rough and smooth towel, a dry and damp one and help put them on the rail. When you are both in the kitchen get him to feel and to taste both hot and cold food. It should be remembered that any child who has problems in feeding usually ends up eating luke-warm or fairly cold food, it is important that occasionally he experiences the differences in temperature or he will become over-sensitive to heat. Let him look into the cupboards, help him open drawers and explore their contents with you, and even tidy up. Fig. 186 shows how it is possible to explore the contents of a cupboard even if sitting balance and mobility are lacking. With a child who is slow to remember and takes a long time to learn and make use of the knowledge he gains – learning in this way is invaluable. It is up to us to see that play is a profitable experience for the child; the presentation of toys is of great importance.

The Moderately Affected Child or the Child who is Beginning to Play by Himself

The *normal* child learns by trial and error – as he plays he experiments. If the cerebral palsied child is to learn in the same way, it is essential that the games played with him and the objects given him are very simple to begin with. If the slightest accidental movement on his part makes an object move or even makes a noise, he will have made something happen himself and this will stimulate him to try again, experimenting on his own, not *directed* to do so. He will have started to learn.

We have found the following useful for simple play:

A large basin of water (in the summer it is better still to put him into the water), see that the objects he has to play with are as varied as possible, heavy ones that sink, light ones that float; things that will make a noise when he bangs them together. Later on use a plastic jug, "Squeezy" bottle, funnel or a colander, all giving a different effect as he takes them in and out of the water. Point out the differences between the objects and the various ways the water pours out of them. Give the child a wooden spoon or soup ladle and saucepan or deep basin, and encourage him to stir or, for example, transfer macaroni pieces or other dry cereals from one bowl to the other. Later, when he becomes more proficient try putting his skill to practical use in the kitchen.

When playing with a hemiplegic child, we have sometimes made the water in a basin of water cloudy in order to stimulate his interest and, in this way, have got him to use his affected hand automatically.

Paper, but *not* polythene, is another simple but enjoyable material for children. A *tissue* square can safely be placed over a child's face to encourage him to blow, or to remove it with his hands. Tissue paper can be made into a ball and pushed up his sleeve or down his vest, it will scratch and make a noise and automatically he will try to see what it is and put up his hands to remove it. All children love balls and paper makes the lightest and safest ball. Hiding a favourite toy in a loose parcel or paper, looking through a hole made in paper, wrap-

231

ping him up in paper, all provide amusement that is sometimes within the capabilities even of the severely handicapped child.

Play-dough or play-foam spread on a mirror, talcum powder on a dark tray, finger-paints, a sand-pit preferably not on legs for the young child, so that he can actually get inside it, and so on, are good ways of enabling the child who has little ability to use his hands and to achieve results, while he plays. A child who seems to have no interest in toys, or in playing with objects around him can sometimes be encouraged at least to look at, or move them away if they are piled on his lap or if he is made to sit on them.

To prevent toys slipping cover the play area with a large 'Dycem' non-slip mat. Where you want toys to move easily over a polished surface, felt secured to the base helps.

The following two ideas are worth trying for the child who frequently drops or throws his toys onto the floor; attach a favourite toy to a belt or to a stout piece of string around the child's waist; or attach a number of different toys or everyday objects to a large cushion.

The Young Cerebral Palsied Child who has the Ability to Balance and to Move

A child who has the ability to balance and to move should *not* play only when sitting in a chair. If he does he will miss the chance of gaining many new experiences. By moving around when at play he will make use of new patterns of movement and acquire new experiences and skills. For example, if he has learned to move from sitting to kneeling upright, place his toys in such a way that he can practise this sequence of movement.

The sketches at the end of this chapter show a variety of ways of encouraging the child to move as he plays (also included are illustrations of play with movement for the more handicapped child, who is still at the stage of being able to use his hands only when sitting), the child should play such games as 'London Bridge is falling down', 'Ring-a-ring o'Roses', 'Oranges and Lemons', and 'Statues', games which will assist in teaching him the concept of 'up and down, round and round' and so on. Obstacle courses are a good way of teaching him to climb over and under, through, sideways and around objects. 'Hide and Seek' is also useful, while the copying of movements in such games as 'Simon says . . .', and getting him to roll over and crawl on verbal command, are all helpful.

It is very important at this stage for the child to become aware of the space that surrounds him as he plays. This should include the space behind him. Encourage him to move in different ways, backwards, forwards and sideways, crawling, upright-kneeling and walking. Games that include throwing a bean-bag over his shoulder or passing a ball over his head, and guessing from a sound behind him what object you are holding, are all ways of encouraging this awareness. Miming to nursery rhymes, conducting or moving to music; playing on see-saws, slides and swings, are ways of playing that will help a child to understand the relationship between space and his own constantly changing position.

Choice of Toys

The following are ideas for simple toys and for play. There are many pre-educational toys on the market; toys such as tricycles, see-saws and so on that can be used only by the *mildly* handicapped child, have been omitted.

Advice on the most suitable toys for a child, according to his age and ability, should be obtained from those concerned with his teaching. No attempt has been made to state any particular age group as so much depends on the ability of the individual child to use his hands, as well as on his level of intelligence, and powers of concentration and comprehension. It is always best to ask the therapists for advice when choosing toys, for in this way you may avoid causing frustration to the child by giving him something too difficult to manage, or else too simple to be a challenge and therefore lacking in interest.

If you are a member of a Toy Library, those running the library will, of course, be able to make suggestions as to the most suitable toys and to give practical advice on the possibilities of each toy; they have also produced an extensive list of toys called the 'A.B.C. of Toys'. Most of the large toy manufacturers now produce excellent catalogues which are clearly divided into various categories, i.e. early stages of play development, indoor and outdoor activities, educational toys and so on, E.S.A. for example, now have a special selection of toys for handicapped children, as a separate section in their main catalogue called 'Play Specials'.

All children love balls. When choosing a ball bear in mind the variety in size, texture and colour that there are; that some are soft and others hard; some have stories in picture-form on them while others play a tune. One can now buy balls that are filled with liquid and have ducks floating inside, others have a butterfly that revolves with coloured beads, both very useful for stimulating the child's interest. A heavy ball, for example, is easier for the ataxic and the athetoid children to play with as their movements are so disorganised and clumsy that the ball is apt to roll away otherwise. A spastic child, on the other hand, can play best with a smaller solid ball as his grip is apt to be too firm and he will have difficulty in lifting a heavy ball. A hemiplegic child should play with a large beach-ball to encourage him to use both hands together. When the child can only grasp a bat or a stick, a ball attached by elastic enables him to play with the ball. For the child who may want to throw and catch a ball but is unable to hold it, a bean bag can be used instead of a ball, this is easy to make and can be made of bright washable material, in many shapes, weights and sizes.

Large wooden light-weight bricks can be used for other games as well as building, i.e. place in plastic bags with coloured or numbered cards and use for matching or grouping. 'Velcro' attached to building bricks will make it easier for the child to build. Bricks are easier to handle than the cards themselves, 'Five-Picture Frame' block for photographs sold by 'Mothercare' can also be used.

If a child has difficulty in playing with his toy cars because he cannot hold onto them, he may manage better if the car is attached to a stick.

If you give a child a toy that requires winding up to make it move, try whenever possible to adapt the key so that he can wind it for himself.

A doll's house made from large wooden boxes is best for the cerebral palsied child, as the 'rooms' will be big enough for him to put his hands inside, and by using larger 'furniture' he will find it easier to move the objects about, see fig. 187 a) b). In a similar way a simple garage can be made at home, see fig. 188.

A toy popular with most children is a 'busy-box'. For the cerebral palsied child a home-made 'busy-box' can be made on a larger scale and designed specially to suit his needs, see fig. 189.

Coloured wooden or plastic cotton reels make excellent counters and can be easily fitted over a board of wooden pegs.

Small empty plastic bottles (make sure that they have contained nothing *toxic*) can be used for guessing games and are a useful size for the child to hold. Fill them with different things to smell and of varying weights and sounds. 'Squeezy' bottles can also be used as a home-made set of skittles.

Most children love music. Listening to the radio or record player is fine but it is far better to encourage them to make their own music. Severely handicapped children, who cannot hold a stick to bang a drum or cannot bang it with their hands, can make a satisfactory noise if a piece of elastic is tied over the top and bottom of the drum. 'Squeezy' bottles filled with sand, buttons, dried peas etc, can give a variety of sound effects when shaken. Bracelets for the wrists and ankles can be made of leather or felt and small bells sewn *securely* onto them, this is a good way to encourage music and movement at the same time. Children love musical boxes, it encourages them to open and close the lid, also encourages the child to put in and take out objects from the music box.

Encourage your child to keep a scrap book. Begin with a room in the house, perhaps, the kitchen. First show and talk to him about the various things found in a kitchen. Then, with him, see if you can spot them in a magazine or paper, and cut them out and paste them into a scrap-book. You can enlarge on this idea when you go out for a walk together collecting leaves, flowers and so on, and pressing them in his book.

When he is beginning to discover that objects have a shape, i.e. round, square, triangular, oblong, collect these with him and then find pictures of them to cut out. Later, the child will get to the stage of copying and drawing the various objects for himself. In this way he will not only learn the names of objects around him but also what they are used for, why they are made in a certain shape, the different colours in which they are made, and so on, see figs. 190 a)–f).

In addition to the toys bought for him, the child usually gets great pleasure in playing with the odds and ends he finds around the house or that he collects in the garden or on his walks. All children are great collectors and hoarders, and if they cannot walk or move around the house they are not only denied the pleasure of exploring and finding out things for themselves, but also of acquiring a private collection of their own. It is up to us if a child is severely handicapped, to take him out to explore his surroundings or bring things to him so that he can find out all about them and keep those he particularly likes. A large magnifying glass is an excellent way of exploring his collection in greater detail, especially interesting if you have been near a pond or river and brought a jar of the water back with you. An outsized magnifying glass with small 'legs' at each corner can be of great interest if placed on the lawn or over a patch of earth.

Poor or clumsy co-ordination of the child's arms, hands and fingers often makes it difficult for him to hold his toys and at the same time to move them around. The simplest way to overcome this is to provide some form of suspension for his toys. For the baby small articles can be threaded on a piece of elastic, ribbon or wool, which can be fastened across his pram or carry-cot; for the older child a bar can be used for heavier toys. The attachment over the table, as illustrated, in chapter 12, fig. 131, is useful since both the distance and the height of the bar can be varied. A bar has been designed to fit across the elevated sides of the cots for *normal* children who are confined to bed, and hanging short ropes on them so that the child can hook his toys upwards within his reach, provides a form of suspension that can easily be adapted for the cerebral palsied child. Be sure to put on the bar a variety of objects differing in weight, size, colour and texture. Toys that the child can safely put into his mouth may be used, *securely* attached to a long piece of string, so that he can gain the experience of feeling them with his lips, chewing and biting them.

When choosing toys do not always go to the toy department in a large store. The kitchen and general sundries department will often have things that can be fun for your child and easily adapted as toys. Shops that sell products from India and Asia have an excellent variety of door-chimes, mobiles, hand-bells and so forth. Craft shops with products from Europe and Russia also have an excellent selection of simple games and toys.

Simple Games using Everyday Things
Many of the everyday objects in the home can, with the application of a little thought and sometimes adaptation, be used in an interesting and amusing way to encourage learning, and at no cost to you.

Take food or soft drink tins or cans, making sure of course, that there are no sharp edges and preferably brightly patterned and coloured ones.

As a moving object often presents a problem for a young child to follow, roll the tin towards him from different angles in the hopes that he will follow it with his eyes, later see if he can push the tin back using both his hands. If an added stimulus is needed, put some dried beans, peas etc., into the tin, the sound will help to attract his attention. Take a number of tins and fill two of each of them with similar objects and by shaking them the child may be able to match similar sounds.

Stick sets of transfers, drawings, cut-out pictures etc., on the lids and inside the bottoms of such tins as those used for tobacco, we have also found margarine cartons useful, and get the child then to match the picture on a lid with the same picture on a base; this is a useful way to teach the child to learn how to match.

Strips of such materials as carpet, emery paper, silk, woollen or fluffy materials when stuck on a tin can be used to help the child to identify the texture of the material by feeling, see that the strips are broad and do not put more than three different materials on one tin. Sew or bind together 5″ squares of knitted material, carpet, curtains etc., then take loose pieces of similar materials to encourage the child to match them.

The shoes and socks of the family can also be used for sorting and pair matching; for the older child folding up dusters, dish cloths etc., and sorting them into appropriate piles is a useful exercise.

Many food packs of the same product can be bought in different types and sizes, some of the lids screw on, others have to be lifted off and so on, these can all be used to encourage fine movements of fingers and hands.

Bowls and containers such as those made by 'Tupperware' are also useful in helping to get fine co-ordination of the fingers, tie pieces of wool, ribbon, string or plastic twine together in a length and put it in the container, then cut a small slit in the lid, pull one end through the slit as a 'starter', and get the child to pull the length through the slit. As it comes through the child should wind it over a stick or something similar – a little competition could be devised to see which of two children can complete the winding over the stick in the shorter time.

An excellent posting box can be made from any square transparent type container as the child can then see what he has posted. Also one can be made from wire-netting so that the child can enjoy the pleasure of watching the pieces as they fall through. The container can be divided into three or four sections with firm pieces of cardboard; apart from posting different shapes the child can be encouraged to fill each section with dried peas, beans, macaroni pieces, different buttons etc. See whether he can name, or even point to the section you name, then let him see what happens when you take away the cardboard divisions and the contents mix, ask him then to try to pick out pieces of similar things.

Children are always fascinated with things that seem to disappear and appear. One way to do this is to take a large *empty* match box, either square or oblong with divisions in it; place different objects in each compartment then let the child open the box by pushing. Another way is to make a hole in the lid of a small cardboard box and another one at the side of the box near the bottom, the child then puts a marble or something similar into the box and then has to shake it to try to get the marble out of one of the holes.

Something that is found in most kitchens – a kitchen plunger with a suction cap – can be used to give a child a lot of amusement while at the same time he learns. By fixing it either perpendicularly or horizontally and using different size rings, the child can be encouraged to stack them on the stick of the plunger, we have found varying sizes of curtain rings useful.

It is hoped that what I have said in the foregoing will be sufficient to prove that the everyday objects in your home can provide many sources of ideas to combine simple play with learning. My experience, with both handicapped and *normal* children, satisfies me that young children get just as much enjoyment, apart from learning value, by the use of the simple things found in their homes. If the child has brothers and sisters they will be ready to offer ideas of their own.

Playing with your Child

Many cerebral palsied children, including the less handicapped hemiplegic children, have difficulty in concentrating and, in our efforts to improve their physical difficulties, we may interfere with and direct their play too much. We all tend to make the mistake, when a child is playing, say, with his bricks, of 'advising' him to 'try the small one on top of the large one', or, when he tries to take the lid off a jar, 'don't pull, turn the lid round and unscrew it'. Then again, as he attempts to push his large model car through a narrow tunnel, 'you will never manage that, try the little car'. The point stressed here is that child will learn far more if he sees the large brick fall off, fails to get the lid off the jar by pulling or fails to push his big car through the tunnel. He should be allowed to make his own mistakes and to reason things out for himself.

He will soon ask for help when he needs it. All this calls for patience. Some children can only manage to play for five minutes at a time, while others play the same game quite happily for twenty minutes. Try always to understand what new things your child is attempting to do and give him the appropriate materials and opportunities, helping him only when he is in real difficulty.

It is most important that we should know and appreciate the maximum amount of concentration a child is capable of giving, for if we ask too much of him he will lose interest and cease to try. Lack of achievement will soon lead to boredom, he will return to the toys and games he knows and understands, and so be deprived of learning and gaining new experiences. The frustration tolerance of a cerebral palsied child is often low, and if he does not succeed at the second or third attempt, he gives up. This applies especially to the child of higher intelligence who knows what he wants to do, but cannot control his muscular reactions sufficiently to allow him to do it.

Children are often easily distracted and it is difficult to hold their attention even for a short time, they soon tire of their toys or games and want to move to something else, with the cerebral palsied child this stage is often prolonged. Here are two suggestions that may help your child to concentrate. When giving him toys offer only two from which to choose, then put away the one he does not want. See that he is not surrounded by things that will distract him, an open toy cupboard, for instance, a pet or other activities going on in the room, playing by the window and so on. He will eventually, of course, have to get used to things going on around him without interruption of his play. When you give the child a new toy, show and explain to him exactly how it works, not once but many times. Stay with him, see if he can manage and that he understands what you have told him, you may find that he would perhaps play better in another position; he may need help to enable him to use his hands, or to be supported to give him better balance. One has to remember that a *normal* child, although he can immediately pick up a new toy and play with it, also often needs quite a lot of help to understand how it works.

Far too often cerebral palsied children, lacking in experience and in imagination, never get past the stage, when playing with cars, for example, of lining them up and then returning them straight to their box, or pushing their trains around and around in the same direction. Help the child to use his imagination by building a garage for the cars so that he can pretend to fill them up with petrol and oil, to wash them and so on, as he may have seen the garage man do. No child learns unless he is interested and it is up to us to stimulate his interest by helping him think of new ideas and situations as he plays. Make sure that it is possible for him to participate actively in the various games, for this is the only way by which he will benefit and learn.

The Play of the Two-year-old Normal Child

Between two and three years of age children as well as playing with their toys begin to be interested in all the things around the house. Anything that Mummy uses or does is fascinating and must be examined and tried. They continually watch and imitate their mother as they play; they want to polish with a duster, to stir with a spoon; to try to wash, dress and undress and take care of their dolls in the same way as their mother looks after them.

Play then becomes more complicated – dolls have tea parties, are put to bed, scolded and praised. If there is a new baby in the house, they are only too anxious to have a live 'doll' to play with, if given a chance. When there are older children in the family they watch and copy them, listen to stories about school and enact the various episodes with their toys.

The Play of the Two to Three-year-old Cerebral Palsied Child

The cerebral palsied child often has the same desire to explore, to find out how things around him work, and to copy and join in the activities of his mother, brothers and sisters, but his handicap prevents him from doing so. If he is to have a chance of enjoying these new experiences, he must be helped. If you are polishing and dusting, give him a duster; even the more severely handicapped child can polish for you as he sits in his chair. The ataxic child who walks in a rather disorganised manner, can help polish the floor if you wrap dusters over his shoes. This should help to improve the co-ordination of movement of his legs, and consequently his balance, as well as giving him pleasure in helping you. A child who drags the toes of his shoes when he walks can be put in charge of cleaning and polishing them, it may encourage him to try harder to lift his feet.

The kitchen is another place where your child can help and learn at the same time. Let him help to cut out some pastry cases, give him something to stir, let him make his own buns, give him the saucepan so that he can put the salt in the potatoes for you. Show and explain to him what you are doing, for example, when you make a cake or sweet, give him some of the ingredients to pour into the bowl or let him help you to weigh them. He will be learning all the time as he watches and helps you to measure, mix and cook. Remember that there will be many questions he would like to ask you, but, either because his speech is poor, or it takes him time to put his ideas into words, he loses the opportunity. A headmaster of a school for handicapped children tells us that often when children are asked at school how pastry is made, they reply 'you get a frozen packet and roll it out', when asked where milk comes from they often reply, 'from a milk bottle'. This is what they have seen, and if they accept the first answer without question, that will be the full extent of their knowledge.

A *normal* child, at about the age of three years, just begins to differentiate between a few basic shapes. He begins by attempting to group together similar shapes, and later at about five years to identify them when asked e.g. which is the circle, the square. He does this by matching shapes, picking one out from a group of shapes, seeing the shape in three dimensions, imitating, copying and finally reproducing the shape when asked.

Difficulty in recognising and differentiating between various shapes and forms is one of the many factors which may prevent the cerebral palsied child from learning to read and to write. It is, therefore, worthwhile spending time in helping the child to feel, to recognise and to match different shapes as he plays. This can be done by teaching him about one shape at a time. Let him really master and understand one shape before introducing another. The following example illustrates how you might do this with a circle; give the child a ball and describe its shape then take his fingers and place them around the ball, letting him feel it in his hands. Let him see, because of its shape, how it rolls, then take a square and show him why, because it has corners it cannot roll. Find objects of the same shape, i.e. different sized balls, an orange, a door knob. Later, get him to make the shape in play-dough or flour dough. You can then show him the round shape in a quoit or other ring and how this circle is a space through which he can see, pass things through, or place over objects. Then point out to him the same round shape in cups, lids, saucers, saucepans. When out for a walk collect some round stones, point out the round of the wheels of the cars and buses, the round flower beds in the park and so on. In this way he will learn to associate a particular shape with many objects, thus extending his awareness of things around him. Place a round sweet amongst some square ones and invite him to find the round one. Later collect together a mixture of round and square objects and ask him to place them into two different groups, then he should be encouraged to make the same shapes with his fingers in sand, flour, with finger-paints, with a pencil or crayons.

All this will be a gradual process taking time and patience, especially when the child has difficulty in using his hands. Continue to persevere, as the learning and understanding of shape is a very important step for many later skills, including reading and writing. Your occupational therapist will analyse the particular difficulties of your child and show you exactly how you can help him.

Later, he will start to place shapes in a simple form board, to make this easier attach handles or knobs to the shapes. These should be of the same colour to begin with, but not too large or they may distort the outline of the shape for the child. Begin by taking one shape at a time out of the board and letting him put it back, then take two, and when he has mastered the three shapes take them all out at once and let him replace them, later turn the board around and ask him to replace the shapes.

Some children find it difficult to grasp and lift an object but are ready nevertheless to learn about the concept of shape and form. A magnetic board is useful for such children, it can be placed flat on a table or propped up in any angle from the perpendicular to the horizontal, or even attached to a peg board on the wall. The makers of magnetic boards also supply figures, letters, shapes and a variety of designs, these are easy for the child to handle as little effort is required to move them around the board. It is now possible to buy magnetic strips for use on a flat magnetic board that can be attached to any toy.

Between the age of three and four, your child may start to be interested in simple jig-saw puzzles. See that his first puzzles are clear simple pictures with a well-defined background and foreground, a picture with too much detail is only confusing for the child. Before he tries to do the puzzle let him really get to know the picture, then take one piece out and let him replace it immediately so that he becomes familiar with each shape. In this way it will be much easier for him to understand how each piece fits the whole.

The visual concept of shape is difficult for many children; the field of perception is a most specialised one and your child's occupational therapist, and later his teachers, will give you expert advice on how to follow up his training. This will include learning how to distinguish between, for example, tall and short objects, a comparison which is often very difficult for the cerebral palsied child who spends so much of his time on the floor or sitting in a chair, and therefore builds up his concept of the size and height of things around him in a limited way. This point has been demonstrated to us even by a child of eleven who, when she stood up for the first time, was amazed to find that the refrigerator, tables and chairs were so much smaller than she had thought.

A child also learns about colour in a definite sequence. First by learning a primary colour, this he will soon recognise, but when shown another colour in comparison he will be unable to identify the second. When he has learned to identify the primary colours he will begin to match similar colours, describing them by name and, finally, naming the colours of things around him.

We hope that in the foregoing it has been made clear how *learning through play* both for the *normal* and the cerebral palsied child, is essential, and that in the process they are being prepared for the basic learning experiences which they will gain when they go to nursery school. Figs. 191 to 214 illustrate some of the ideas which will help to utilise the child's 'play activities' as a means of progress towards independence and as the basis for future learning. Figs. 215 to 220 illustrate some of the problems and suggestions for play specifically for the hemiplegic child.

At this point I must draw attention to the correct way to use the large beach ball I referred to in this chapter and to the rolls and rollers which have been frequently mentioned.

The use of large beach balls and rolls and rollers as aids in treatment, and later for play, originated during my work at the Western Cerebral Palsy Centre.

Looking at the sketches of the beach ball and the roller an impression might be formed that they were intended to be 'soft', whereas, in fact, the ball must be fully inflated and the roller kept fairly firm.

It is important to remember that each of these items is used to encourage balance and righting reactions and that a firm base is essential if the child is to have sufficient extension in combination with rotation – the basis of future balance.

A soft ball, whether the child lies on his tummy, back, or leans over it while standing, will merely result in increased flexion and is completely *ineffective and useless*.

It is most important when using any type of equipment to be clear in your mind as to why you chose it in the first place and to make certain that the child not only benefits generally by its use, but that he also acquires a skill which before he had found to be impossible.

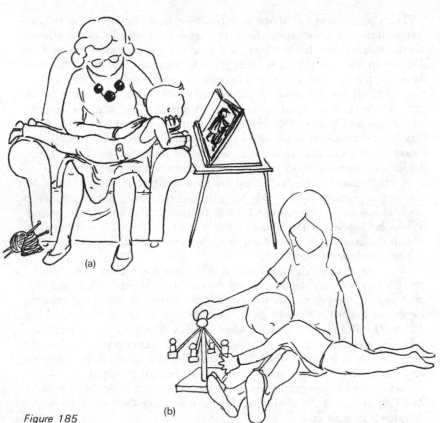

(a)

(b)

Figure 185
(a) The child lies on his tummy supporting himself on his arms. His grandmother helps him to straighten his back and applies light pressure under his chin to enable him to hold his head up.
(b) His teen-age sister takes a turn to play with her brother. Growing more accustomed to lying on his tummy and with fewer spasms the child can lie on the hard surface of the floor and no longer needs help in holding his head up.

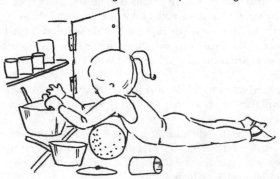

Figure 186. By using a roller in this way the immobile child can enjoy exploring the contents of a cupboard

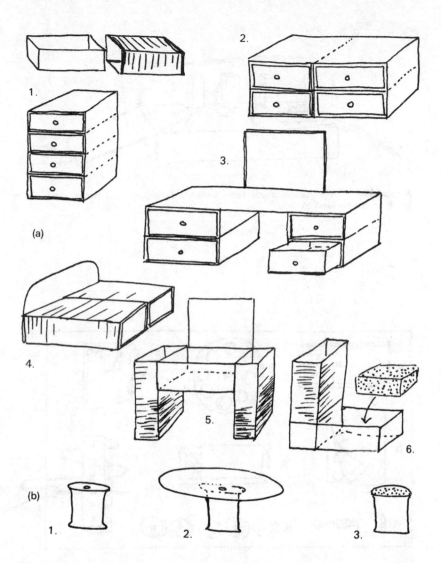

Figure 187. All matchbox furniture can be covered with adhesive paper or other adhesive material.

Mirrors can be made of plain cardboard covered with aluminium foil.

a) 1. Chest of drawers (upright) – 4 whole matchboxes covered.
  2. Chest of drawers (side by side) 4 whole matchboxes covered.
  3. Dressing table – 4 whole boxes with cardboard top and mirror.
  4. Double bed – 2 matchbox covers, headboard, covered with material.
  5. Washbasin stand – 1 inner box, 2 matchbox covers, with mirrors.
  6. Chair – 1 whole matchbox, a piece of foam in the base for padding covered with material or cotton wool.
b) 1. Cotton-reel as a base for 'furniture'
  2. Circle of cardboard glued to top of a reel forming a 'table'.
  3. Small circle of foam attached to reel forming a 'stool'.

243

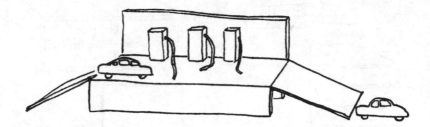

Figure 188. Petrol Pumps made from wooden blocks – feed hoses made from piece of cord nailed to side.

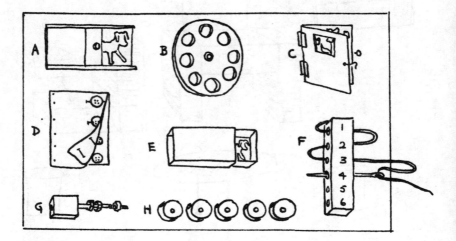

Figure 189. Busy Box.
A. Sliding door – or small runners with a picture behind the door.
B. Telephone dial.
C. Hinged door – with hook fastenings, photograph or child's own drawing pasted inside.
D. Material with buttons – inside is a felt head of a flower or butterfly attached by a popper to the material.
E. Match box – filled with a series of small cards or small buttons, etc.
F. A threading block – very popular with most children.
G. Large bolt mounted horizontally on block with screwing nuts.
H. Removable cotton reels fitted on pegs with corresponding colours or corresponding numbers.

244

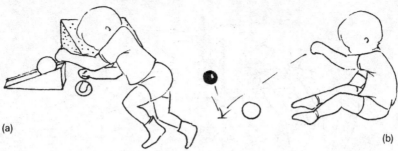
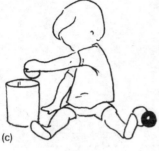
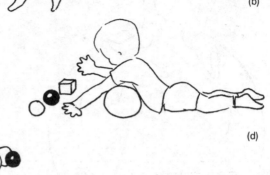
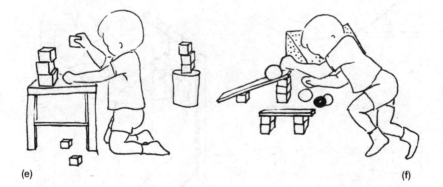

Figure 190. Learning basic perception from balls and blocks for children with limited ability.

(a) Provide a ball to roll, feel etc.

(b) Introduce more balls – soft, and of hard-wood rubber etc.

(c) Drops in container for sounds.

(d) Introduce a block with the balls – to discover difference in feeling, purpose – block cannot roll.

(e) Remove balls – introduce more blocks – child learns about building towers, bridges etc.

(f) Replace balls with blocks and experiment possibility of complementing each other e.g. make ramps with blocks to roll balls down, build towers for balls to knock down etc.

245

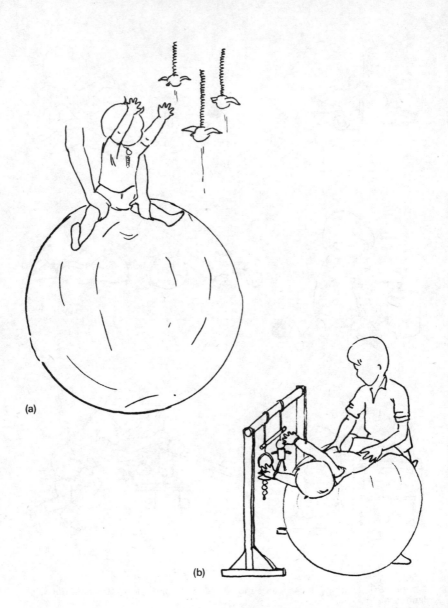

Figure 191
(a) Sitting on the ball, as illustrated, is a useful preparation for the *spastic* child who finds it difficult to sit in long-sitting on the floor; movements sideways, backwards and forwards will encourage balance and adjustment of the position of the head, if his trunk is rather *floppy*, bumping him on his bottom will help give him stability.
(b) Child playing on his back on the ball to encourage rotation with the head and arms forward, a movement he will need to roll over and sit up.

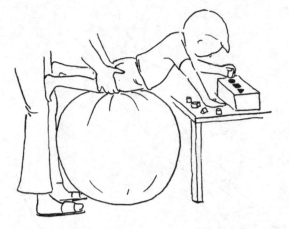

Figure 192. For the child who finds it difficult to lift his hands and his back when he lifts his arms forward to play, lying on his tummy on a large ball as illustrated, is useful to get this combination of movements. Keep the hips and legs straight and turned out, watch to see that the feet do not get stiff, with the toes pointed downwards. Some children have legs that part too easily, if so, keep them together. If you want rotation of arms and trunk and sideways movement of the head move the ball slightly sideways.

(a) His feet are flat against his mother's legs. As the posting box calls for accuracy and fine finger movements, the child is allowed to support himself on one arm.

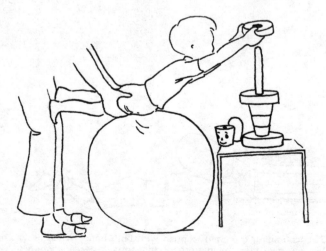

(b) Firm inhibition and stability is given at the hips and pelvis to encourage the child actively to extend.

247

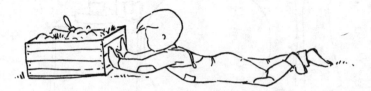

(c)

(c) The most advanced position as extension against gravity at this angle is difficult especially when using the hands in this way.

Figure 193. Encouraging the child to push with both hands while he lies on his tummy. This will give him the pattern of the arms necessary when using his hands, e.g. for supporting himself or protecting himself when he falls.

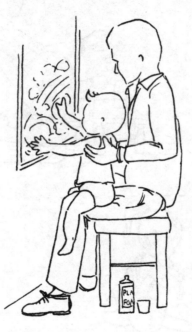

Figure 194. Child sitting astride his father's knee makes shapes out of play-foam on a mirror. His shoulders are lifted up and pressed forward to help him give pressure with his hands.

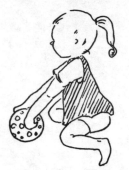

(a)

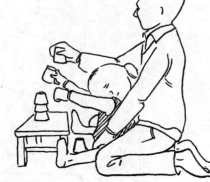

(b)

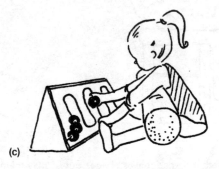

(c)

Figure 195
(a) Typical abnormal position of a *spastic* diplegic child, sitting between her legs which are turned in at the hips. Because of her wide base in this position she can balance and her hands are free for playing.
Continually sitting in this way, will in time cause flexor contractures of hips and knees.
(b) Child sits well forward at the hips, legs straight and turned out, in some cases control at the knee is preferable. Check continually to see that his hips are really bent and that he sits symmetrically.
(c) The first step towards sitting on her own can be achieved by placing a roll horizontally over both legs, just above the knees. The child keeps both arms forward over the roll which helps her keep her hips bent and legs straight.

250

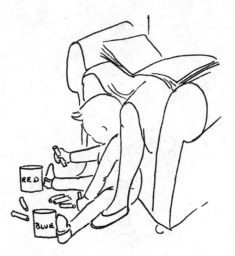

Figure 196. The child plays on the floor. His mother controls him at the shoulders with her legs and at the same time provides stability at the hips with her feet.

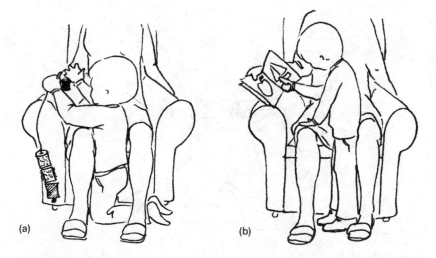

(a)

(b)

Figure 197
(a) The child maintains an upright position being controlled between his mother's legs. He is threading cotton reels covered with different materials, e.g. sandpaper, fluffy material, paint etc.
(b) The child stands supported by his mother's legs. He is looking at a book with simple bold pictures – tracing around the picture with his finger – while mother says – 'take your finger up, around, down, under, across, the middle' and so on.

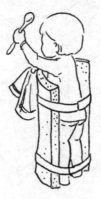

Figure 198. Young mildly affected child plays in standing; the foam 'case' is used to give confidence rather than support, strips of 'Velcro' hold foam together. The toy illustrated is suspended to encourage him to lift his head and arms, helping him to stand up straight. The top of the case prevents the child from pressing his arms down.

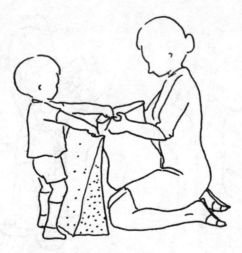

Figure 199. Child supports himself holding on to foam wedge. Mother holds bag with such objects as comb, brush, spoon, cup, apple, pencil, sock: the child guesses *without* seeing what is in the bag, purpose is tactile perception.

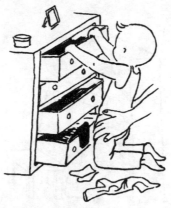

Figure 200. Playing in kneel-standing position – keeping the hips straight and weight on both knees. If the child is rather 'wobbly' at the hips give pressure down as illustrated.

(a)

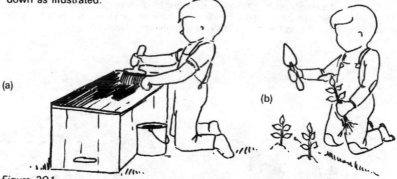

(b)

Figure 201
(a) Washing and painting a large wooden or cardboard box using a painter's brush. The brush is easy for the child to hold and encourages him to make large sweeping movements.
(b) Making use of upright kneeling while putting plants in the garden.

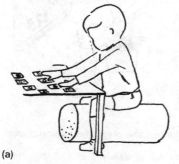

(a)

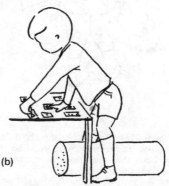

(b)

Figure 202
(a) A roller with a low table in front encourages the child to move from sitting to standing while he plays.
(b) The child in the illustration is matching up cards.

253

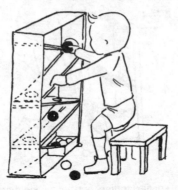

Figure 203. A simply constructed 'ball run' to encourage play at different height levels, or use a cabinet with drawers at different levels. As the child explores you can get him to stop at the height he finds most difficult, or slowly get him to move up and down as he plays with the different levels of drawers.

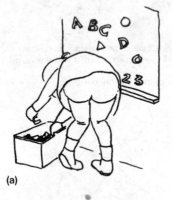

(a)

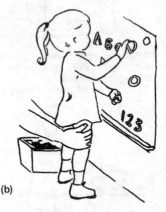

(b)

Figure 204. To prevent the child becoming stiff when she plays in standing, place the things she is playing with on the floor.
(a) Note that the effort of bending down causes the legs to turn in and the child to go up onto her toes.
(b) To stop this abnormal pattern, hold at the knees or high up on the thighs turning them out and see that the weight is well forward. Tell the child to straighten her legs. Maintain this control as she bends down to get another letter from the box.

254

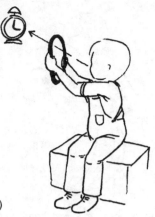

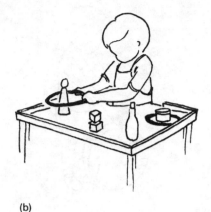

(a)

(b)

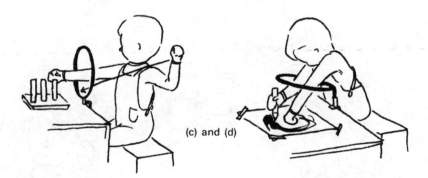

(c) and (d)

Figure 205. Play that needs good co-ordination between eye and hand when *sitting.*

(a) The *athetoid* child finds it difficult to grasp while he holds his arms steady and particularly difficult to keep his head still and look at what he is doing. When he first plays as illustrated, you may have to hold his feet down for him.

Using the ring as a camera and focusing it on different objects in the room. For the older child you can play 'I Spy' in this way.

(b) Placing a ring over an object without touching it. A number of rings can be used and care must be taken to see that no ring touches the other.

(c) and (d) A ring clamped on the table as illustrated can be used if the child cannot use his hands, because his arms keep 'flying' outwards.

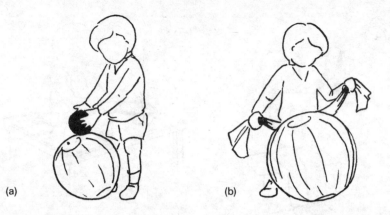

Figure 206. Play that needs good co-ordination between eye and hand when *standing*.
(a) Balancing one ball on another, using only the fingertips, then slowly moving the ball forward with the legs, while the small ball remains on the top.
(b) Moving a ball in all directions as the child walks about guiding it with a towel held in both hands.

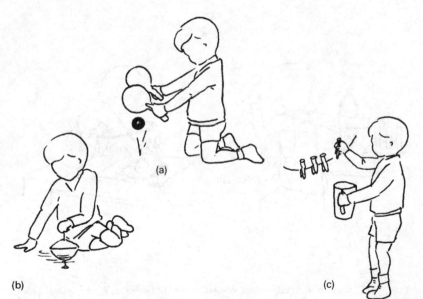

Figure 207
(a) Playing with two bats; lifting, bouncing and catching a ball. In the illustration the child grasps with the whole hand; if the index finger is held straight along the back of the bat the movement used will be a good preparation for writing and eating with a knife and fork.
(b) Working mechanical toys such as a humming top.
(c) Movements that involve holding with one hand while we move the other, come into all our functional activities – leading to the hardest of all-doing different movements with each hand.

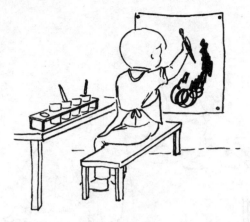

Figure 208. By placing the stool next to the wall, as illustrated, and attaching a large piece of paper to hardboard or a blackboard, the child has to rotate his body as he paints; this is good for his head and trunk control.

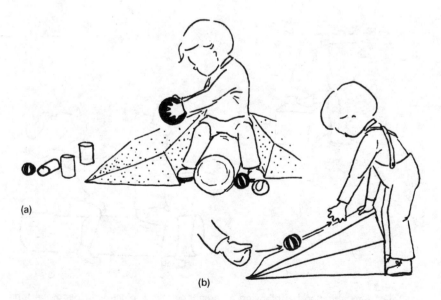

(a)

(b)

Figure 209. Activities that encourage movement and eye-hand control.
(a) Sitting.
(b) Standing.

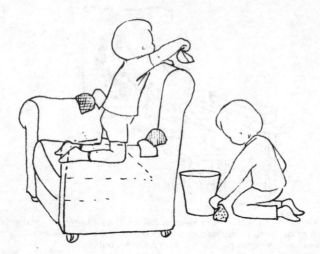

Figure 210. Using the back of the chair for upright-kneeling – throwing bean-bags into a bucket, combines movement and eye-hand control.

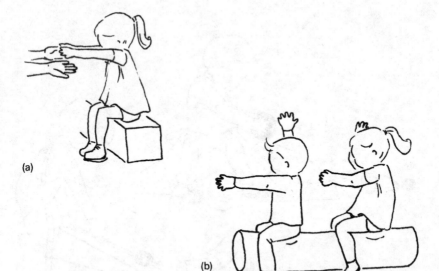

(a)

(b)

Figure 211
(a) Illustrates imitation by following a verbal command 'place your hands on top of my hands' – 'underneath my hands' and so on.
(b) Imitation by copying. Child sits directly behind a *normal* child, later and more difficult facing another child or adult. Encourage the child to describe his actions 'what am I doing' – 'what are you doing'.

258

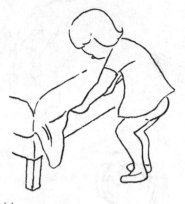

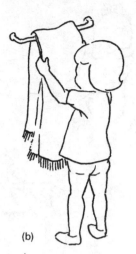

Figure 212. Two-handed activities.
(a) Holding, pulling and pushing
(b) Folding and placing over rail

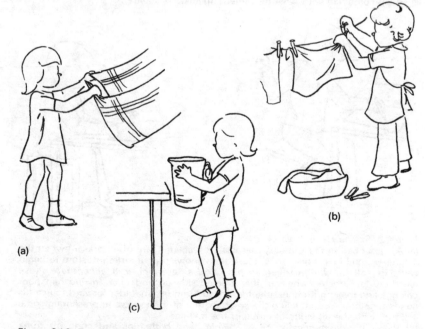

Figure 213. Two-handed activities.
(a) Shaking and holding
(b) Finger-thumb opposition, placing pegs on a line.
(c) Holding weight, lifting and pouring.

259

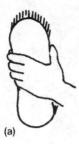
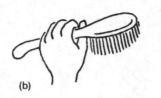
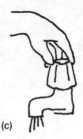

(a)
(b)
(c)

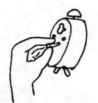
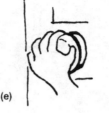

(d)
(e)

Figure 214. One-handed activities.
(a) Open handed grasp.
(b) More refined grasp.
(c) Finger-thumb opposition.
(d) Finger-thumb opposition – finer co-ordination.
(e) Grasp combined with wrist movement against resistance.

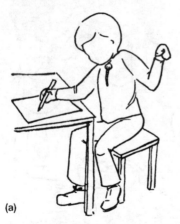
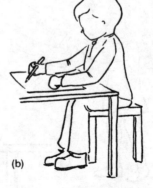

(a)
(b)

Figure 215. The Hemiplegic child.
(a) As described in the Glossary 'associated reactions' are often present when the *hemiplegic* child uses his hands, illustration shows a poor sitting posture to begin with, i.e. all his weight over on his good side which will *accentuate* these reactions, pulling the whole of the affected side up and back, giving him poor balance and making it impossible for him to bring his shoulder forward to use his hands together. Also affecting the co-ordination of the eyes, and presenting some children with the difficulty of crossing the mid-line.
(b) By sitting symmetrically, he is able to bend both hips and bring his trunk forward. The 'associated reactions' will still be present, but he has a better chance to keep his shoulders forward and therefore a greater possibility of using both hands, and to have better eye-hand co-ordination.

260

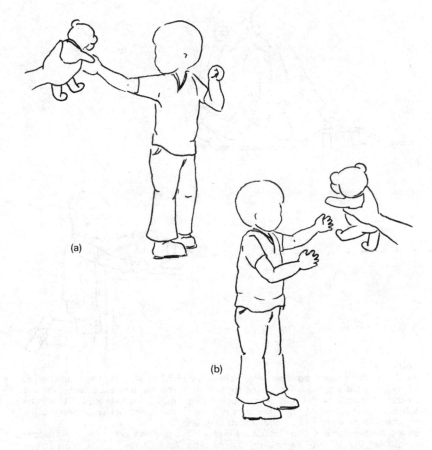

Figure 216
(a) When you hand toys or objects to a *hemiplegic* child it is important to take trouble to see that you are directly in front of him. If you stand, for example, on his unaffected side, as illustrated, you can see how the abnormal patterns of the whole of the affected side are reinforced, even the head is pulled more towards this side as the child looks and reaches out for his teddy bear.
(b) If handed to him in mid-line and slightly to the left he becomes more symmetrical.

261

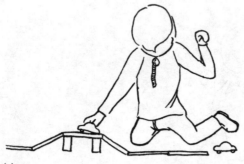

(a)

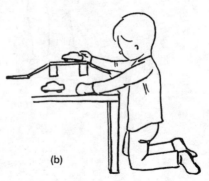

(b)

Figure 217
(a) This is *not* a good position for a *hemiplegic* child to play in. He is inclined to sit on his good leg, his affected leg turning in at the hip and knee with pressure on the inner side of the foot. The affected (left side), in our sketch, of the trunk is bent, the shoulder of his flexed arm is pulled down and back. He cannot bring his shoulder forward to use both hands together.
(b) Kneel-standing is a good position for play. This position helps the child to take weight equally on both legs, with straight hips. As he uses his hands he has to balance, making adjustments in his whole body. Playing in this way will help to improve his standing balancing and therefore his walking.

262

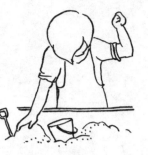

(a)

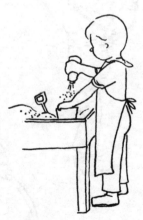

(b)

(c)

Figure 218
(a) Illustrates the strong 'associated' reactions often found in the affected arm of the *hemiplegic* child when using his good hand.
(b) Stop this reaction by turning the arm out and up at the shoulder keeping the elbow straight, the hand is held with the thumb out, when possible also extend the wrist.
(c) The child is encouraged to keep his affected arm forward supporting himself on his opened hand. Note the sandpit is at waist height enabling the child to stand straight.

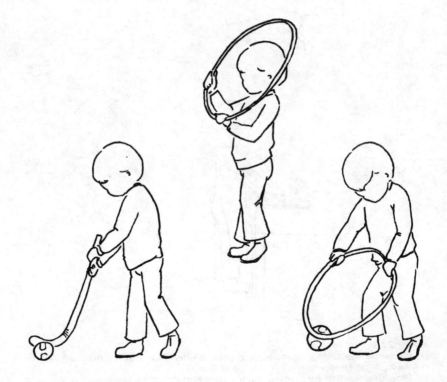

Figure 219. If the *hemiplegic* child, unless he is helped by you, can only hold a ball as illustrated it is better to give him a stick, bat and ball, or hoop and ball to play with.

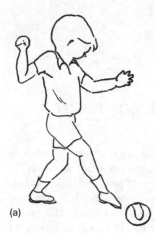

(a)

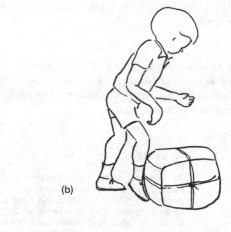

(b)

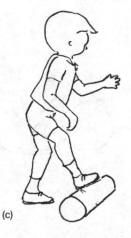

(c)

Figure 220
(a) It is not a good idea to encourage a *hemiplegic* child to kick a light small ball; unable to stand on his affected leg he will kick the ball as illustrated, leaning his body backwards, increasing the stiffness in his leg and the bending of his arm.
(b) Kicking a parcel or medicine ball which gives resistance, is good exercise for the child. He moves the parcel or ball while his leg is bent, his body-weight coming forward.
(c) The child moves the roller by pushing it along with his heel.

EARLY STAGES OF NORMAL DEVELOPMENT

The posture of the normal baby for the first few months is predominantly one of flexion. At this early stage his head is rarely in mid-line, he has no active head control other than the ability, when placed on his tummy, to turn his head sideways to breathe. His arms are usually bent with loosely closed hands, his legs bent and apart. His 'mass' movements are abrupt and follow no set pattern. He reacts to light and to loud sounds by blinking or by a Moro reaction, neither stimulus having any meaning for him.

STAGE ONE
The first significant stage in motor development is that of mid-line orientation and the start of head control. Both of these activities make it possible for the baby to begin to make contact with his environment, first with his eyes and much later as he explores with his hands.

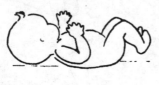

Figure 221
(a) Supine
At this stage the baby prefers to lie on his back. His head is now usually in mid-line. He brings his hands together over his chest, and looks at them. This combination of touch and vision is the first important step in self-exploration. He takes his hands to his mouth, at first accidently and then purposefully to suck, later touching and exploring his lips, cheek and tongue with his fingers. His eyes start to co-ordinate and he becomes pre-occupied with his mother's face, but to begin with only at mother-to-child distance of 6''.

(a)

Rolling
For the first time the baby starts to move from one position to another, he does this by rolling to either side from his back. To begin with he will often hold his hands together while he rolls. The movement of rolling starts with the turning of the head which causes the body to follow (neck-righting reaction) later the baby initiates the movement himself.

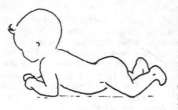

(b)

(b) Prone
Head control starts to develop first when the baby lies on his tummy. It should be noted that the top of the spine extends sufficiently to enable the baby to get his shoulders and arms forward. Weight is taken on the forearms which help him raise the upper part of his body. His hands remain loosely closed; one often sees the baby scratching the surface with his fingers.
The pelvis which was previously up in the air when lying on his tummy is now flat on the support, his hips and legs are bent and apart, feet dorsi-flexed.

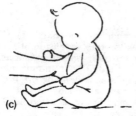

(c)

(c) Sitting
At this stage the baby must be supported when sitting. He holds his head erect but only for a few seconds. Even though his back is straight *except for the lumbar region* his body has to be supported in sitting long after he has complete head control in this position. His arms and legs are bent and abducted, feet dorsi-flexed.

Vision and the beginning of eye-hand regard

Gradually the baby starts to select what he sees, he can follow his mother as she moves around the cot, follow a simple dangling toy 6″ to 12″ above his face through a half circle from side to side.

He begins to turn to the sound of a voice, smiling when his mother speaks to him. He is already learning to smile when he wants to be picked up, and to know that if he cries he will get attention.

STAGE TWO

The next important pattern of motor development is the beginning of extension-abduction of the limbs (overlapping with flexion abduction) in conjunction with the extension of the whole body. He practises this extension in all positions but at the same time is able to do activities in flexion.

Figure 222

(a) Supine

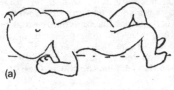

Illustration (a) is one of many ways by which the baby practises extension when lying on his back. In the sketch his shoulders are retracted arms bent, hands loosely closed. His feet are flat on the floor and he lifts his bottom off the support. In no time he will learn to push himself back in this way. He also has the ability to *lift* his head *forward* despite the fact that his shoulders are retracted.

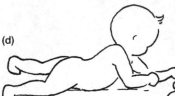

(b) We have included this sketch to illustrate that although so much time is spent practising extension, the baby is *also* able to bring his arms *forward* to place his hands on his bottle. Hand regard – playing with his hands and fingers and taking them continuously to his mouth – is a very important part of learning at this stage.

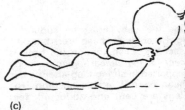

(c) Prone

We can see in this sketch how the 'high lifting' of his head facilitates the total extension of his body, including for the *first time the lumbar spine*. He lifts his arms either bent and off the support as shown in the sketch, or off the support with his arms extended sideways. The term 'swimming on his tummy' is often used to describe this activity.

It is important to note that although his legs are lifted and extended they are apart and the feet remain dorsi-flexed.

(d) We include this sketch to illustrate that the baby can *also* at this stage take weight on his forearms and reach out to touch a toy. His feet are dorsi-flexed and toes bent pressing against the floor, later he will use this position of the feet when he starts to creep.

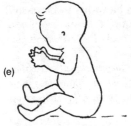

(e) Sitting

The baby's head is now steady, his body straighter including, for the first time, the beginning of *extension in the lumbar spine*. His arms are bent, abducted and retracted at the shoulders, or forward as shown. His legs are bent and apart, feet dorsi-flexed. It is at this stage in his development that we often find it difficult to bend the baby's hips to sit him. He enjoys pushing himself back when in this position, he still needs support.

Vision and the beginning of eye-hand co-ordination

The baby can, as it were, now 'grasp' an object with his eyes but is still *unable* to reach out and grasp it with his hands. He shows excitement and the fact that he wants something by kicking with both legs and waving both arms, *opening and closing* his fingers as he does so. At first he does this with his arms bent and near his body, but gradually progresses to opening and closing his hands as he both follows and reaches out for the object – but he is still unable to grasp or to manipulate at this stage. It is worth noting that this is the first time that we see the baby making a deliberate attempt to move his arms *towards* an object with the intention of trying to get it.

He can follow an object if it is moved slowly from left to right in front of his face. If we place a rattle in his hand he grasps it strongly with the inner side of his hands and fingers. He can look at it for a *second* and then starts to wave his arms about in an unco-ordinated way, often hitting himself and complaining loudly – *he cannot at this stage let go* (rattles are so varied in shape and sound these days that they are an excellent way of trapping the ears and eyes at this stage of development).

Hearing and Speech

He responds momentarily to loud sounds, vocalising as he moves and answering back in his way to sounds made by adults, in conjunction with the variation of pitch his repertoire enlarges, for example sounds of anger appear. He blows 'raspberries', syllables come into his babbling and he starts to make the sounds 'm' 'mm' and 'ddd'.

STAGE THREE

The baby has progressed from being a flexed to being an extended individual and now he has perfect head control. He has now reached the *important stage in his development when he starts to break up these total patterns and a greater variety of motor patterns appear. This is the stage of strong extension – abduction of the limbs.* Where before movements of the limbs were taking place predominantly at the shoulders and hips, we now see active movements appearing at the elbows and knees. It should be noted that the development of the arms is still in advance of that of the legs.

Rolling

He can now roll over from his tummy onto his back, a movement that includes *rotation* and active extension of the whole body, so essential when he finally stands and walks.

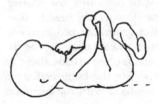

Figure 223
(a) Supine
At this stage the baby starts making movements for a desired result, for example he reaches out with his arms when his mother approaches to pick him up. As the baby reaches out with his hands he has his hips bent and often his legs straight, a pattern he will use when getting up from sitting, and when he sits with his legs straight out in front. This pattern of reaching out is a very important one coinciding as it does with his ability to grasp. He now finds his feet for the first time, and is able to integrate his ability to see, feel and grasp by holding onto his feet, becoming aware of how they look, both when still and when moving; he furthers his knowledge of himself by taking his feet to his mouth.

(a)

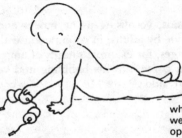

(b) Prone
When on his tummy the baby not only raises his head high with a completely straight back, but whereas a few weeks earlier he was taking weight on a closed hand, the hand is now open. Because of the mobility of the arms, when using them for support, he is very soon able to take his weight on one arm and reach out for his toys with the other — forward and later behind him.

(b)

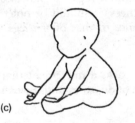

(c) Sitting
He sits now with his legs apart and straight out in front of him, his feet are dorsi-flexed. He has no sitting balance, still tending to throw himself backwards when sitting. Because of lack of sitting balance and the lack of support sideways, he is often apt to fall over sideways. He begins to use his hands for support at this stage, but *only* in front of him.

(c)

270

Vision and Manipulation

As head control is now complete the baby can follow objects with his eyes in all directions, he is also able to fix his gaze on small objects. Where before when seeing his image in a mirror he was puzzled, he is now aware of himself and will reach forward and pat his image. Self exploration is now complete as the baby goes a step further and becomes aware of his feet.

Object exploration begins as he now has developed the ability to look, reach, touch and clutch an object with his whole hand. Manipulation is still very crude and for this reason everything is immediately taken to his mouth, the mouth playing an important part in providing information such as taste, shape and consistency.

He still has no fine movements of his fingers; flapping and scooping with his hands, having to open the whole hand widely before grasping and succeeds in this way in picking up, for example, a 1″ wooden cube. His grasp is a 'palmar' one, i.e. with the whole hand. Movements at the wrist are becoming noticeably more refined. He can hold and transfer two cubes of 1″, but if he drops one he *takes no notice*. He will accept large objects with both hands, looking at them and immediately taking them to his mouth. Wooden spoons, bricks and cups are much preferred at this stage to soft toys.

Hearing and Speech

He now turns immediately to sounds *except for* those that come from directly above his head, which tend to confuse him. He responds when spoken to by laughing, chuckling and squealing, vocalising with variations in a tuneful way. The continuous sounds he makes are forerunners of future speech, his babbling is repetitive using syllables such as 'ppp' and 'sss'.

STAGE FOUR

The baby now reaches the stage in his development when *his ability to rotate becomes well co-ordinated.* Whilst rotation was present before when he rolled, reached across for an object when lying on his back, or when lying on his tummy supporting himself on one arm as he reached back with the other, now with arm support sideways developing as well as forwards, *spontaneous rotation, trunk control and sitting balance appear.*

Rolling

He now rolls from his back to his tummy in a well co-ordinated manner where previously he was rather disorganised.

271

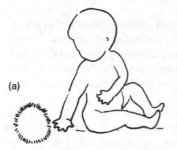

Figure 224
(a) Sitting to prone
He now uses his ability to support himself on one hand, pushing himself up to sitting at the same time as he rotates his body and vice versa. He pivots on his tummy, also pushing himself backwards, the legs remaining rather inactive at this time, another example of how the development of the arms is still in advance of the legs. Later he will creep forward, his legs participating strongly in the movement, especially the feet.

(b) Sitting
At first unsupported sitting is of short duration, probably no longer than a minute, the baby will then lean forward to support himself. With the gradual development of trunk control and sitting balance he learns to support himself sideways. Arm support is first done with a loosely closed hand, later the hand opens in preparation for bearing weight.

Vision and Manipulation

As we have already pointed out a baby's ability to reach and grasp objects is dependent on his balance and his ability to look at what he is doing. It is therefore not surprising at this stage, to find him making exaggerated movements of his whole body and often over-balancing in his attempts to reach out for a toy. During the following months these exaggerated movements gradually diminish.

His ability to manipulate improves rapidly at this time, his grasp becoming more refined, he can now hold one object in each hand and transfer from hand to hand and bang two cubes together. He starts to take objects *out* of a container and tries unsuccessfully to pick up small objects. He starts to 'drop' large objects onto the floor, a basic pattern for future release, but once they have been dropped he has no further interest in them.

Speech

He uses sounds to express his anger and hunger and 'n-n-n-n' sounds to express dislikes and imitates dialogue using chains of sounds with intonation.

STAGE FIVE

The final developmental stage we shall deal with is the *acquisition of balance and the beginning of progression*. Most activities at this time start from the sitting position, moving around is the most important function for the baby at this stage – an opportunity to start exploring his environment and himself in relation to his environment.

Supine

On the rare occasions when he does lie on his back he does so now with his legs straight and slightly apart.

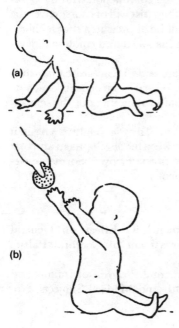

(a)

(b)

Figure 225
(a) Crawling position
As we stated at the beginning of this section, moving is of prime importance at this time. The baby now only plays for short periods on his tummy, preferring to get on all fours where he rocks in preparation for crawling, a movement that requires both balance and reciprocal movements of the legs.

(b) Sitting
Backward protective extension of the arms is now starting. He has good balance in sitting and no longer relies on his hands for support. As illustrated, he can turn to look and grasp a toy with good rotation of the trunk, or alternatively pivot in the sitting position.

Eye-hand development

At this time *isolated movements* of the fingers are possible enabling him to explore objects with his finger tips and poking them with his index finger. The *thumb and index finger* now play an important part in manipulation, small objects being picked up and inspected. It is important to note, at this stage, that although manipulation has now reached a more advanced stage, release of an object is still impossible, the baby attempts to release by pressing an object against a surface. Play now is more purposeful and the baby becomes engrossed for longer periods at a time, he is becoming aware of the permanence of objects and when he drops a toy on the floor will *look to see* where it is gone.

Speech

He vocalises deliberately as a means of communication and understands the words 'no' and 'bye-bye' and enjoys copying adults, for example, when they cough.

NOTE. Whilst obviously there are other stages in the motor development of a *normal* child during the period we have covered here, such as getting up to sitting, sitting to standing, standing to walking, I have confined this Appendix to the most important early stages to provide examples of how the gross motor patterns of movement in supine, prone and sitting underlie the fine motor skills of the hands; I have taken these on conjunction with the development of vision, hearing and speech; your therapist will of course cover the whole of the matters in greater detail. It will be appreciated that a child's ability to learn at different stages, including his social and emotional development, is of equal importance.

The purpose of this Appendix is to illustrate and to emphasise that when we are helping the cerebral palsied child towards independence in any functional skill it is essential that we understand something of the sensorimotor patterns that underlie these skills.

Given this understanding of the development of a *normal* child as a basis, it will be easier to understand the differences between his development and that of the cerebral palsied child, enabling us to appreciate how abnormal movement patterns interfere with future achievements.

References

BOBATH B. (1971): 'Motor Development, its Effect on General Development, and Application to the Treatment of Cerebral Palsy'. *'Physiotherapy' Journal.*
SHERIDAN M.D. (1960): 'The Developmental Progress of Infants and Young Children'. Reports on Public Health and Medical Subjects. No. 102 (1969).

Appendix II

QUESTIONNAIRE

This is a copy of the questionnaire used at the Child Development Centre, Charing Cross Hospital. Adequate space is provided on the form in which parents, with the help of the occupational therapist, put their answers.

GENERAL
Give names and ages of any other children in
the family.

Has he had, or is he having any therapy

Has your child had any operations, plasters, or
any modifications to his shoes

Has your child been prescribed drugs; if so,
give the reason, type and dosage

Has he had his hearing and vision tested
If so, by whom, when and where

Does he attend a dentist regularly
Give the name and address of dentist.

Is your child at
    (a)   Day Nursery
    (b)   Nursery School
    (c)   Playgroup
    (d)   Baby-minder
    (e)   At home with you at all times

If other than (e) above, how many daily hours
attendance are spent away from home; give the
name and address of place and of person
in charge.

If you have put your child's name down for
school when he is five years old, state name and
address of school.

FEEDING

Does your child eat with the family.
If he can feed himself are there still times when
he demands that you feed him.
Does he drool
  (a) when eating
  (b) when sucking a sweet
  (c) when making sounds.

Are there any of the following difficulties when
feeding. If so, describe:
  (a) tongue thrust
  (b) gagging
  (c) continual sucking
  (d) inability to close mouth when feeding
  (e) swallowing
  (f) biting immediately something is placed
      in his mouth
  (g) biting off a piece of food
  (h) chewing.

If you have to help your child with his feeding,
what position do you have him in whilst
feeding him.
Does he need a special chair.
Describe the type of general control you
provide.
Describe the specific help given to the jaw, lips
and tongue to enable him to chew and swallow.
Is he hypersensitive to having a spoon put in
his mouth.
If so, what does he do.

Can he feed himself with bread, biscuits, or any
other food with his hands, or do they crumble
in his hands.

Can he feed himself with
  (a) a spoon
  (b) with a fork
Which hand preferred.
How does he hold these –
  (a) with a fist
  (b) between thumb and fingers.
Do you you have to help him get food off his
plate. Can he take food up to his mouth, or
does he have to take his head down towards his food.

Does he bring his spoon straight towards
his mouth or sideways.
Does he have any difficulty in closing his lips to
get the food off a spoon or fork.
Does he do this with his teeth or lips.
Can he manage together
    (a)   spoon and pusher
    (b)   spoon and fork
    (c)   knife and fork.
Can he cut up his own food.

Does he have difficulty with certain foods.
Indicate those that are impossible, hard
to manage, or disliked:-
    (a)   liquids, hot or cold; ice cream.
    (b)   crisp foods, e.g. cereals, raw vegetables,
          toast, biscuits.
    (c)   slippery foods and eggs.
    (d)   sticky foods, e.g. bacon, meat, chicken.
    (e)   sipping and chewing, soup with
          vegetables etc.
    (f)   large bites and chewing, e.g. apples.
Are there any foods not listed that are
especially difficult.
Does he have food fads.

Are there difficulties when your child drinks. If
so describe what you do to help him. Do you
have to pour liquids down his throat with his
head backwards.
Does he drink from a bottle, straw, Polythene
tube or a special cup with a spout.
Does he try to hold his cup or mug with one
hand or both.

SPEECH
*The following questions apply only to a child who
has difficulty in speaking:*
When your child was a baby did he make
noises in his cot. If so describe them.
Does he understand when you speak to him or
do you have to use gestures.
Does he respond to his name and look around
when you call him.
Does he seem to listen to you when you speak
to him. How does he show his interest, i.e. stop
what he is doing; look at the person speaking.
How does he behave if you cannot understand
what he is trying to tell you.

Does he make any sounds either in response to
your voice or for his own pleasure. Describe

briefly what he does.
Does he put sounds together, e.g. 'Da-da', 'Ba-ba'.

How does he make his likes, dislikes and needs
known to you, e.g. when wanting the lavatory,
a drink, a toy out of reach etc. –
  (a) by facial expressions
  (b) by gestures
  (c) by sounds.

Has he a way of indicating 'Yes' or 'No'.

Give examples of the type of words
  (a) he can manage
  (b) he finds difficult or impossible
  (c) does he rely on gesture.

Does he use a word or words with a particular
reference to a person or object.
  When you ask him to fetch something does
he respond, or appear not to understand
your request.

Does the effort of speaking make him go stiff
or result in involuntary movements.
Is his ability to use his hands affected when
he speaks.

When does he use language most frequently
  (a) with parents
  (b) with other children.

Does he join in with songs, nursery rhymes, etc.

CARRYING
How do you carry him.

Do you have any difficulties when you
  (a) pick him up
  (b) when you are carrying him.

Does he stretch his arms out towards you to be
picked up.

278

PRAMS AND CHAIRS
What type of pram or push-chair have you.
What type of chair and table does he have,
describe any modifications or adjustments made.

Describe what difficulties he has when he sits
on the floor or in a chair, does he
  (a)   tend to fall to one side; if so, which
  (b)   slide forwards
  (c)   push back
  (d)   Can he place his feet on the support
  (e)   find it impossible to use both hands
        together when in a chair without arms.

MOVEMENT
Does your child move by
  (a)   rolling (to which side)
  (b)   push himself around on his back
  (c)   creeping, crawling, shuffling along on
        his bottom
  (d)   walking along the furniture
  (e)   walking independently.

Does he fall often, bump into people or objects.
Find difficulty in going through a doorway.

Can he manage stairs – up and down.
  (a)   crawling or walking
  (b)   two feet to a step or alternating his feet
  (c)   does he have to hold on.

Can he walk in the street without holding your
hand. If not, by which hand do you hold him.

Can he get on and off kerbs.

Does he tire quickly when out walking.

Does he have a special walking aid. If so, does
he use it inside/outside the house or both.

Does he have – a tricycle, bicycle, scooter or
pedal-car.

What adjustments or modifications have been
made, if any, to the above items of equipment.
Can he get on and off them without help.

_____

Does he go to the swimming baths, horse-ride
or take an active interest in any other outside
activities.

_____

WASHING
Do you wash your child in the family or baby bath.

_____

Do you have any difficulty with his balance in the bath.

_____

Does he sit or lie.

_____

Does he fall over when you wash one leg.

_____

Does he co-operate when you bath him.

_____

Does he need any type of bath aid e.g. rubber
ring, non-slip mat, special seat.

_____

Can he get in and out of the bath.
What help does he need.

_____

Can he wash and dry his hands and face.

_____

If yes, does he do so sitting or standing at a basin.

_____

Can he turn the taps on and off.

_____

Can he put in and pull out the plug.

_____

Do you brush his teeth, or does he do so himself.

_____

Is an ordinary or electric toothbrush used.

_____

Can he squeeze the toothpaste.

_____

Can he rinse out his mouth.

Can he brush his hair.

Can he comb his hair.

Do you have difficulty in washing his hair,
if so please describe.

TOILET
Is he clean and dry
   (a)   during the day
   (b)   at night.

Does he wear nappies or trainer pants.

When did you start potty training.

Does he have a special 'potty-chair'.

Can he sit safely on the pot or toilet.

Can he manage his toilet by himself.

If not, how much help do you have to give him.

If he suffers from constipation what do you do.

SLEEPING
At what time does your child go to bed/get up.

Does he have a rest during the day.
When and for how long.

Does he have difficulties going to sleep.
Is he a light sleeper.

Does he wake up and cry. If so, how often.

Does he want to come into your bed during the
night, if so, do you allow this.

Does he sleep with his head back, mouth open.

Does he move in his sleep or do you find him
in the same position.

Is he uncovered in the mornings.

Do you have to turn him.

Can he cover and uncover himself and turn in bed.

Can he get in and out of bed himself.

Does he have a cradle over his feet at night.

Describe what, if any, adjustments you have
made to the cot or bed.

DRESSING

In which position do you dress your child
if he is a baby or unable to help himself.
  (a) On his tummy, back or side
  (b) On your lap, on a table
  (c) Sitting or standing
  (d) Do you use different positions for
        various garments.

Are there garments (including nappies), with
which you have any particular difficulty
  (a) Putting on
  (b) Taking off.

Do you speak to your child about the task in
hand while dressing him.

Does your child co-operate
  (a) Lift his arms, his leg, give his foot etc.
  (b) Push his head through his t-shirt,
        arms through sleeves, etc.

282

When trying to undress or dress himself, does
your child sit on the floor, or on a chair, or stand.
Or does he use different positions according to
the clothes he is putting on or taking off.
Describe.

Which clothes can he
  (a) Take off
  (b) Put on

Can he manage
  (a) Buttons, back, side, front, on cuffs
  (b) Laces, buckles
  (c) Back fastenings
  (d) Zips
  (e) 'Velcro'
  (f) Press studs
  (g) Hooks and eyes
  (h) Tie.

Is he aware that his clothes have a
  (a) Left and Right side
  (b) back and front
  (c) inside and outside
  (d) top and bottom
and apply them correctly when dressing.

BEHAVIOUR

Is he a happy child – does he have mainly
'good' days or 'bad' days.
How does he behave when
  (a) cross
  (b) shy.

Is he
  (a) calm, placid or very active
  (b) shy or clinging.

When he has been naughty and you are
displeased does he understand.
Are you as firm with him as you are with your
other children (or as you think you ought to be).

Does he get jealous if not the centre of attention.
If there are other children in the family, are they
apt to spoil him, letting him have his own way.
Does he dislike being with other people without you.

Do you have any special difficulties with your child
when in public, e.g. street, shops, restaurants.

Does he understand danger.

Does he have any special fears.

PLAY
If a baby, does he play 'peek-a-boo', 'pat-a-cake', wave 'bye-bye',
join in nursery rhymes with actions. Describe.

Does he take toys to his mouth
  (a) always
  (b) sometimes
  (c) not at all.
Does he look at toys you hold or place in front of him.

Does he reach out for toys.

Does he have a preference for one hand.

Does he use both hands when playing.

How long are his play sessions.

How does he like to amuse himself most.

Does he play the same way with the same
things each time. Describe.

Does he chatter as he plays.

Is he constructive or destructive in play.

In which positions does he find it easiest to play
  (a) Lying on his tummy or side
  (b) Sitting on the floor, or on a chair
  (c) Squatting or kneeling
  (d) Or, has he no particular preference,
        moving about as he plays.

What type of toy does he prefer.

Does he have a special favourite.

How does he play with them, e.g. move, bang,
build or throw them on the floor.

Can he screw, unscrew, put things in and out
of a container.

Can he build, horizontally, vertically.

Does he push and pull toys.

Is he interested in picture books.

How does he look at them, i.e. quickly turning
the pages, slowly asking about the pictures.

Does he draw or paint, with or without instruction.
Describe.

Does he play in an imaginative way, e.g. tea parties,
dressing up, washing and putting dolls to bed.

Is there any kind of experience that he particularly enjoys,
e.g. music, a colour, being taken out in a push-chair.

What type of toys or objects around the house
does your child prefer to play with.

Does he 'help' with the household duties or
imitate you while dusting, cleaning the shoes,
laying the table and so forth. Give examples.

Will he play alone.

Does he have the chance to play with other children.

Does he like their company, or prefer to play
alone with you.

Does he play better with his brothers and sisters
than with other children.

When with other children does he play with or
alongside them.

Does he enjoy any special activity alone with his father.

Does he have his own special pet at home,
does he look after it himself.

Can he play on a slide, swing, climbing frame
or see-saw. If there are difficulties, describe.

Is there one particular aspect of your child's
behaviour or management with which you feel
we can help you.

GLOSSARY FOR PARENTS

The terms we use

Abduction: movement of the limbs away from the midline of the body.

Active movements: movements a child does without help.

Adduction: movements of the limbs towards the midline of the body.

Agnosia: loss of ability to recognise experiences from the special senses (e.g. visual and auditory) and from other parts of the body, e.g. touch.

Aphasia: inability to perform purposeful movements although there is no muscular or sensory loss or disturbance.

Associated reactions: increase of stiffness in spastic arms and legs resulting from effort.

Asymmetrical: one side of the body different from the other – unequal.

Ataxic: a type of cerebral palsy in which the child has no balance, he is jerky and unsteady, his movements are poorly-timed, graded and directed.

Athetoid: a type of cerebral palsy in which the child has uncontrolled and continuously unwanted movements.

Atrophy: wasting of muscles or nerve cells.

Automatic movements: necessary movements done without thought or effort.

Balance: maintaining equilibrium.

Body awareness: knowledge of one's body – in terms of both the idea of its different parts and their relation to one another.

Cerebral Palsy: disorder of posture and movement resulting from brain damage.

Clonus: shaking movements of spastic muscles after the muscles have been suddenly stretched.

Colour Perception: the recognition and differentiation of hues and intensity of colour.

Contracture: permanently tight muscles and joints.

Contralateral: refers to the opposite side, usually concerns extremities, e.g. right arm, left leg.

Co-ordination: the patterning of the action of the muscles of the body, i.e. their 'working together' is controlled by the brain and is necessary for the maintenance of posture, for balance and the performance of movements.

Cyanosis: blue discoloration due to circulation of imperfectly oxygenated blood.

Deformities: body or limbs fixed in abnormal positions.

287

Development: growth of the brain and body.

Developmental Dysphasia: delayed development of normal language and speech due to neurological damage.

Diplegia: a type of cerebral palsy the legs being mostly affected, but often with some involvement of the arms.

Distractable: unable to concentrate.

Dorsi-flexion: the lifting of the foot up towards the body.

Dyslexia: impaired ability to read.

Equilibrium: state of balance.

Eversion: turning out of the foot.

Extension: straightening of any part of the body.

Eye-motor co-ordination: the ability to co-ordinate vision with motor activities.

Facilitation: making it possible to move.

Flexion: bending of any part of the body.

Flaccid: floppy –(see Hypotonia).

Floppy: loose or poor posture and movements.

Hypotonia ('Floppiness'): decreased muscle tension, preventing maintenance of posture against gravity, also difficulty in starting a movement due to lack of fixation.

Handling: holding and moving with or without the help of the child.

Head control: ability to control the position of the head.

Hemiplegia: a type of cerebral palsy in which only one half of the body is involved. It is usually this type of child who shows asymmetry most clearly.

Inhibition: a technical term used in treatment. Special techniques of handling are aimed at stopping the spastic or athetoid patterns which prevent or interfere with normal activity.

Inversion: turning in of the foot.

Key points: parts of the body mostly proximal from which one can reduce spasticity and simultaneously facilitate more normal postural and movement reactions.

Movement: change of position.

Monoplegia: a type of cerebral palsy in which only one limb is affected – rarely seen.

Muscle tone: the state of tension in muscles at rest and when we move – regulated under normal circumstances sub-consciously in such a way that the tension is sufficiently high to withstand the pull of gravity, i.e. to keep us upright, but it is never too strong to interfere with our movements.

Nystagmus: continual oscillation of the eye-balls.

Occupational therapy: treatment given to help the child towards the greatest possible independence in daily living.

Passive: that which is done to the child without his help or co-operation.

Pathological: abnormal.

Patterns of movement: in every movement or change of posture

288

produced by it, the brain throws muscles into action always in well co-ordinated groups that is in patterns.

Perception: the process of organising and interpreting the sensations an individual receives from internal and external stimuli.

Perseveration: unnecessary repetition of movement and/or speech.

Phonation: ability to utter vocal sounds.

Physiotherapy: the treatment of disorders of movement.

Planta-flexion: the pointing of the foot downwards.

Posture: position from which the child starts a movement.

Primitive movements: baby movements.

Pronation: turning of the arm with palm of hand down.

Prone: lying on tummy.

Quadruplegia: a type of cerebral palsy in which the whole body is affected.

Reflexes: postures and movements completely beyond child's control.

Retardation: slowing down of physical and mental development.

Righting: ability to put head and body right when positions are abnormal or uncomfortable.

Rigidity: very stiff posture and movements.

Rotation: movement that takes place between hip and shoulder or vice versa.

Sensori-motor experience: the feeling of one's own movements.

Skill: ability to perform a task.

Spasm: sudden tightening of muscles.

Spasticity: stiffness.

Spatial: relationship of one thing to another in space learned through vision and movement.

Speech therapy: treatment given to develop and to improve speech, and to help with feeding problems.

Stereognosis: the ability to recognise shape, size and/or weight of objects.

Stimulation: provide the desire to move, speak, etc.

Supination: turning of the arm with palm of hand up.

Supine: lying on back.

Symmetrical: both sides equal.

Tonic neck reflex: when the turning of the head causes one arm to straighten and stiffen and the other to bend and stiffen.

Trunk: the body as distinct from the limbs.

Valgus feet: flat feet.

Visual memory: the ability to retain and reproduce shapes seen briefly.

Voluntary movements: movements done with intention and with concentration.

SUPPLIERS OF EQUIPMENT AND ACCESSORIES

PUSH CHAIRS

The Baby Buggy
Measurements 3′ 5″ × 6½″ × 6½″.

The Buggy Major
Measurements 107 × 19 × 16.5 cm. (3′ 6″ × 7½″ × 6½″).
Obtainable from: The Spastics Society and through a doctor's recommendation by the Department of Health & Social Security. Also obtainable from Mothercare and Boots.

The New Anyway with accessories
Obtainable from: Mothercare.

Li-Bak Folding Push Chair with hood and apron
Obtainable from: Boots Chemist and the manufacturers, Cindico Ltd, Skerne Road, Driffield, North Humberside.

Meyra Pushchair (Erwin)
Obtainable from: Meyra Rehab UK, Millshaw Park Avenue, Leeds 11.

Insert Seat
Obtainable from: Cindico Ltd, Skerne Road, Driffield, North Humberside.

CHAIRS

The 'Bean Bag' Chair
In three sizes – in washable cotton with a zip or in 'BUKFLEX' (polyurethene fabric) easily washable with a cloth or sponge.
Obtainable from: Mrs. S. Armstrong, 8 Irving Road, London W.14 or Mrs. S. Rice, 120 St. Stephens Avenue, London, W.12.

'Safa' Bath Seat
Obtainable from: The Spastics Society.

Baby Relax Seat Seven-in-One
Can be used as low or high chair or potty chair.
Obtainable from: Leading stores or the manufacturers – Baby Relax Ltd., 113 Wennington Road, Rainham, Essex.

Baby Relax T.V. Chair
Child's plastic and steel-framed chair, similar in design to the 'Cosco Go-Go' chair.
Obtainable from: Leading stores or the manufacturer – Baby Relax Ltd., 113 Wennington Road, Rainham, Essex.

'Star Rider' Car Seat
Recommended for use in home as described in the Chapter on Chairs, for children between 10 months and 4½ years. The firm has also produced a safety harness.
Obtainable from: Mothercare and many large stores.

KL Jeenay Safety Seat
Recommended as a safe car seat – see magazine 'Which' for tested car seats.
Obtainable from: Manufacturers K.L. Automotive Products Ltd., 25/37 Hackney Road, London, E.2 (approved B.S.I.) and from many large department stores.

Saddle Seat Engine and Desk
Obtainable from: E. J. Arnold, Parkside Lane, Dewsbury Road, Leeds LS11 5TD.

Corner Floor Sitter with Tray and Accessories
Obtainable from: Rifton, Robertsbridge, East Sussex.

Toddler Chair
Obtainable from: Rifton, Robertsbridge, East Sussex.

Adjustable Corner Seat with Tray Fitment
Obtainable from: Nomeq, Washford Mills, Ipsley Street, Redditch, Worcestershire.

Folding Canvas Corner Seat (folds 61 × 41 cm: sides 40 × 38 cm).
Obtainable from: Nottingham Medical Aids, 17 Ludlow Hill Road, Melton Road, West Bridgford, Nottingham.

The 'Mountain Chair'
Obtainable from: E.S.N. Aids.

Theramed Chair
Obtainable from: Theramed Chairs, Theramed Ltd., P.O. Box 57, Camberley, Surrey.

Potty Chair
Obtainable from: Mothercare.

Pete Chair – Ladderback
Obtainable from: Contacting The Spastics Society and Athletic Equipment Manufacturing Co. Ltd., Brantham Mill, Berhgolt Road, Brantham, Manningtree, Essex CO11 1QY and Sherwood Industries, Rainworth, Nr. Mansfield, Nottingham NG21 0HW.

Chunky Chair
Obtainable from: E. J. Arnold, Parkside Lane, Dewsbury Road, Leeds LS11 5TD.

Seat for Unsteady Children
Obtainable from: ECKO Plastics Ltd., Southend-on-Sea, Essex.

Bath Seats
Obtainable from: Orthokinetic (U.K.) Ltd., 24 South Hampshire Industrial Park, Totton, Southampton.

Bath Chair (small and large)
Obtainable from: Rifton, Robertsbridge, East Sussex.

Bolster Chair
Obtainable from: Rifton, Robertsbridge, East Sussex.

FEEDING AND DRINKING

Beaker tyle mugs
'Doidy' cup (Polypropylene) especially recommended for small athetoid children.

'Teacher' beaker non-tip – for children with no head control – slow flow.

Small two handled slant mug with lid (type with 2 holes in lid recommended only).

'Tommie' Tippe Cup
Obtainable from: Most leading chemists and many large stores.

'Rigidex' two-handled beaker (polythene)
Capacity three-quarters of a pint. Height 4", size of handle 3½". Recommended particularly for the athetoid child.
Obtainable from: The Spastics Society.

Wine-makers Wide Tube (cannot be chewed)
Obtainable from: Boots Chemists.

Plates

Divided Warm Plate
Obtainable from: Mothercare.

Keep Warm Plate
Obtainable from: Mothercare.

Keep Warm break resistant divided plate.
Obtainable from: Most leading chemists and many large stores.

Non-slip Mats
'Dycem' plastic can now be obtained in rolls of varying widths – this material is easy to cut.
Obtainable from: Nottingham Medical Aids, 17 Ludlow Hill Road, Melton Road, West Bridgford, Nottingham.

Foam filled plastic covered mats
Obtainable from: Mothercare and Simplantex.

Suction Egg Cup
Obtainable from: Homecraft Supplies, 27 Trinity Road, London, S.W.17.

Bibs

Long-life Dikky bib
Obtainable from: Mothercare.

Absorbent Terry Bib with waterproof backing, ties at waist for extra safety.
Obtainable from: Mothercare.

Absorbent Terry Coverall Bib with waterproof backing.
Obtainable from: Mothercare.

FOR BUILDING UP HANDLES OF CUTLERY

'Rubazote' Tubing
Obtainable from: The Spastics Society.

Plastazote Tubing (hardwearing)
6 ft (1.8 m) lengths.
Obtainable from: Nottingham Medical Aids, 17 Ludlow Hill Road, Melton Road, West Bridgford, Nottingham.

Plastic Wood (tube or tin)
Obtainable from: Most hardware stores.

Cutlery
Sunflower Ultralite Lightweight Cutlery with easy grip handles.
Obtainable from: Nottingham Medical Aids, 17 Ludlow Hill Road, Melton Road, West Bridgford, Nottingham.

BATHING

Safa Bath Seat
Obtainable from: The Spastics Society.

Bath Mats (non-slip)
Baby's Safety Bath Mat. Size 17" × 10".
Toddlers Safety Bath Mat. Size 22" × 14".
Obtainable from: Mothercare.

Liquid bath cleansers for severely handicapped children to replace soap.
Obtainable from: Mothercare, Boots and other large stores.

Towels with shaped hoods
Obtainable from: Mothercare and other large stores.

Bath Seats (for older children)
Obtainable from: Orthokinetics, 24 South Hampshire Industrial Park, Totton, Southampton.

TOILET

Potties
Mothercare Potty (polypropylene with wide firm base)
Mothercare Toddler Training Seat
Obtainable from: Mothercare.

'Watford' Potty Chair (made of wood, safety bar across front)
Size 17″ high, 12″ base, seat 9″ square.
Obtainable from: The Spastics Society.
No potty supplied: Halex No. F501 will fit this chair – obtainable
from retailers.

Baby Relax Toilette
Obtainable from: Baby Relax Ltd., 113 Wennington Road, Rainham,
Essex, also from many large stores.

Large Nappies
Size 30″ × 30″ and 36″ × 36″.
Obtainable from: The Spastics Society.

Mothercare Selection of Nappies
Nappy liners and disposable nappies
Shaped terry napkins

Tuffty Tails
Obtainable from: Most chemists.

SLEEPING

Drop Sided Cots
Choice of two mattress heights.
Obtainable from: Mothercare.

Baby rest-sleeping bag, in shower proof quilted nylon with warm
lining. Can also be used in Baby Buggy.
Obtainable from: Mothercare and Simplantex.

SHOES

Shoo Shoos
'La Parisette' Shoo Shoo Bootees, all leather, open to the toe, visible
fittings style 6229 sizes 2–7 including ½ sizes. White only.
Obtainable from: F. E. Abbott & Co. Ltd., 104 Homerton High Street,
E9 6JG.

Remploy Bootees, all leather, open to toe, sizes 2–8.
Obtainable through: Doctors recommendation and prescription and
from the Department of Health and Social Security.

Pedro Boots
Obtainable from: Gilbert & Melhuish, 503 Bristol Road, Birmingham
B29 6AU.

White Open Toe Sandal (Bata), also **Clark's Sandals**
Obtainable from: Children's shoe departments at large stores and most
large shoe shops.

Wellington Boots in PVC with Warm Lining
Sizes 4, 5, 6, 7, 8, 9, 10 with short or higher leg.
Obtainable from: Mothercare.

Odd shoe list
Obtainable from: The Spastics Society; this list gives the name of shops
who are willing to supply odd shoes for children.

For reinforcing toe caps

Shoe Guard
Obtainable from: Howmedica International Ltd., 622 Western
Avenue, Park Royal, London, W.3.

Shoe Plastic
It is advisable from time to time to write to the Spastics Society to see
if any new material for reinforcing toe-caps has come on the
market.

BOOKS

Books for Babies
Pictorial Folding Book (Galt's & Heal's stores).
'I see a lot of things'. Published by Collins.
'First things'. Published by Collins.
Minibooks. Published by Methuen.

Simple Picture Books for Very Young Children
Topsy and Tim series – Published by Blackie.
Ladybird Picture Book Series.
Blackie's 'Chunky' series e.g. 'My Teddy'. Published by Blackie.
'Things we do' and others by Dean Hay – Published by Collins.
'Toddle About' (folding books) e.g. 'Come into the Town'. Published
by Young World Publishers.

Activity Books
Ladybird Play Book 1–4.
'Not Yet Five' – ideas and suggestions for the pre-school child.
Activity Colouring Book. Published by Collins.

Nursery Songs & Rhymes
'This Little Puffin' – Penguin Pocket Book.
The Oxford Nursery Song Book.

Books for the 2–5 year olds
Beginning Beginners Series, e.g. 'The Foot', 'The Eye', 'The Ear',
books. Published by Collins.
'Inside, outside, upside down.' 'Hand, hand, fingers, thumb.'
Published by Collins.

'Fun to Sniff' book – Published by Hamlyn London Books.
'Paul in Hospital'. Published by Methuen.
'Play in Hospital'. Published by Faber & Faber.
'Give your Child a Better Start'. Published by Cressels Publishing Co. Ltd.
'A Playschool Beginner Book'. Published by World Distributors (Manchester).

Books with good illustrations and stories of everyday activities enjoyed by the younger child
'A book for me to read' series. Published by Bancroft.
'Breakthrough to reading' series. Published by Penguin. e.g. 'My Mum', 'The Loose Tooth'.

Books with good pictures for slightly older children
Richard Scarry's 'Best Word Book Ever'. Published by Hamlyn London Books.
Althea Series, e.g. 'George the Baby' – Published by Dinosaur.
Dick Bruna Series, e.g. 'My Vest is White'. Published by Methuen.

Reading guides for different age groups
Obtainable from: The Children's Book Centre, 140 Kensington Church Street, London, W.8.

Children's records
Kiddicraft Series.
Number Rhymes.
Action Rhymes.
Singing Games.
Obtainable from: leading record stores.

Books on Toy-making
'Do-It-Yourself Toys'.
Obtainable from: The Toy Libraries Association.

Making Music with the Handicapped Child by Elaine Streeter. Published by C. Steers, 150 Railway Terrace, Rugby, Warwickshire.

The Human Horizon Series. Published by Souvenir Press Limited, 43 Great Russell Street, London WC1B 3PA.

Parents Information Bulletin – Mental Handicap. *Obtainable from:* The Bookshop, NSMHC Centre, 117 Golden Lane, London EC1Y 0RT.

Getting Through to Your Handicapped Child, by Elizabeth Newson and Tony Hipgrove. Published by C.U.P.

Therapy Through Play, by Ivonny Lindquist. Published by Arlington Books, London.

Helping the Retarded: A systematic behavioural approach, by E. A. Perkins, P. D. Taylor, A. C. M. Capie. Published by B.I.M.H., Kidderminster, Worcs.

MISCELLANEOUS

Alarm Systems
Obtainable from: Mothercare and Boots Chemist.

Mod Baby Rocker (bouncing cradle)
Obtainable from: Mothercare and Boots Chemist.

Hammocks
Obtainable from: Large stores, babies and children's departments.

C.P. Steerable Walker (data sheet Part No. 96-00)

Circular Walker (De Luxe)
Obtainable from: Baby Relax Ltd., 113 Wennington Road, Rainham, Essex.

The Cheyne Nursery Walker
Obtainable from: Pryor & Howard Ltd., Willow Lane, Mitcham, Surrey.

Triangle of the 5-piece Variplay Triangle Set
(can be used as a baby walker)
Obtainable from: Community Playthings, Robertsbridge, East Sussex.

C.P. Prone Tricycle Mk. 2. Adjustments 8 parts (information sheet No. 23).
Obtainable from: Rehabilitation Engineering Services.
Ontario Crippled Children's Centre, 350 Rumsey Road, Box 1700, Postal Station "R", Toronto 17, Ontario M4G 1R8, Canada.
NOTE The above firm do not have manufacturing facilities for general use, but may be willing to make a few special orders available to competent centres on special order. Prescriptions **only** accepted from professional persons in the field of celebral palsy.
The following designs from the above although not mentioned in this book may also be of interest.
A Saddle Walker.
Choice of three 'wheeled base'.
Stroller base for small children, Mooney Base for older child who cannot propel himself, Wheelchair base for the older child who can – or who may learn to propel himself.

Tiny Trike
Obtainable from: James Galt and Company Ltd., Brookfield Road, Cheadle, Cheshire.

Mobility Trike
Obtainable from: Tri Aid Manufacturing Ltd., 29 James Watt Place, College Milton North, East Kilbridge, Lanarkshire.

Munster Horse
Obtainable from: Everest and Jennings, Princewood Road, Corby, Northants.

Adjustable Canvas Wedges
Height at front Min. 20 cm. Max. 30 cm.
Length Min. 53cm. Max. 76 cm.
Width 50 cm.
Obtainable from: Nottingham Medical Aids, 17 Ludlow Hill Road, Melton Road, West Bridgford, Nottingham.

Foam Wedges
8½″ at apex tapering down to a point.
24″ wide, 25½″ long.
Wedges should be covered with a washable material or terry towelling.
Obtainable from: The Spastics Society.

Also available are foam wedges that have been sprayed with plastic, providing a washable hard surface.

Prone Board (prone-scooter boards)
Obtainable from: Rifton, Robertsbridge, East Sussex.

Small Prone Stander
Obtainable from: Rifton, Robertsbridge, East Sussex.

Flexistand
Obtainable from: Joncare, Meadjess Ltd, Radley Road Industrial Estate, Abingdon-on-Thames, Oxon.

P.V.C. Play Therapy Balls
80 cm and 110 cm.
Obtainable from: The Spastics Society.

Baby Carrier (cuddle up)
Obtainable from: Boseywear Ltd., 36 Keswick Road, High Lane, Stockport, Cheshire.

Reversible Cot Bumper Velbex covered.
Obtainable from: Mothercare.

Electric Toothbrushes
Obtainable from: Most leading chemists.

Adaptive Easel
Obtainable from: Rifton, Robertsbridge, East Sussex.

Reeves Clever Crayons triangular crayons.
Obtainable from: Reeves and most large stores.

Stirex Scissors
Obtainable from: Nottingham Medical Aids, 17 Ludlow Hill Road, Melton Road, West Bridgford, Nottingham.

Therapy Swing
Obtainable from: Rifton, Robertsbridge, East Sussex.

Bolster Swing
Obtainable from: Rifton, Robertsbridge, East Sussex.

Foam Ramps
Obtainable from: Rifton, Robertsbridge, East Sussex.

Diffraction Box
Obtainable from: Huntercraft, Ramsam Stable, Priestlands Lane, Sherborne, Dorset.

Fiddlesticks
Obtainable from: Huntercraft, Ramsam Stable, Priestlands Lane, Sherborne, Dorset.

Special garments – range of garments specifically designed for play clothes for the C.P. child.
Obtainable from: The Spastics Society.

Polystyrene beads bags of 12 cu ft.
Obtainable from: Mrs. S. Armstrong, 8 Irving Road, London, W.14.

ADDRESSES OF GENERAL INTEREST

Toy Libraries Association, Seabrook House, Wyllyotts Manor, Darkes Lane, Potters Bar, Herts. (Tel: Potters Bar 44571).

Disabled Living Foundation, 346 Kensington High Street, London W14 8NS.

The Spastics Society (Head Office), 12 Park Crescent, London W1H 4EQ.

The Spastics Society (for information and equipment), 16 Fitzroy Square, London W1P 5HQ.

Royal Society for Mentally Handicapped Children and Adults (MENCAP), 123 Golden Lane, London EC1Y 0RT. (Tel: 01-253 9433).

Riding for the Disabled Association, Avenue "R", National Agricultural Centre, Kenilworth, Warwickshire CV8 2LY. (Tel: 0203 56107).

The National Association of Swimming Clubs for the Handicapped, 219 Preston Drive, Brighton, Sussex BN1. (Tel: 0273 59470).

ASBAH (Association for Spina Bifida and Hydrocephalus), Tavistock House North, Tavistock Square, London WC1 9HJ. (Tel: 01-388 1382).

Break, 20 Hooks Hill Road, Sheringham, Norfolk NR26. (Tel: 0263 823170). Holiday and short stay centre for handicapped children.

Calibre, Aylesbury, Bucks HP20 1HO. (Tel: Aylesbury 32339). Cassette library for blind and handicapped children.

Cheyne Holiday Club for Handicapped Children, 61 Cheyne Walk, Chelsea, London, S.W.3. (Tel: 01-352 8434).

Deaf Children Society, National, 45 Herefore Road, London W2 5AH. (Tel: 01-229 9272).

National Society for Epileptics, Chalfont Centre, Chalfont St. Peter, Bucks SL9 0RJ. (Tel: 02407 3991).

Special Care Centre for Families, Sunley House, 10 Gunthorpe Street, London, E.1. (Tel: 01-247 1416). Services for handicapped children and parents.

Kith and Kids, 27 Old Park Ridings, Grange Park, London N21 2EX. (Tel: 01-360 5621).
Self help group for parents with a handicapped child.

Pre-School Playgroups Association, Alford House, Aveline Street, London SE11 5DJ. (Tel: 01-582 8871).

Voluntary Council for Handicapped Children, National Children's Bureau, 8 Wakley Street, London EC1V 7QE. (Tel: 01-278 9441).

Special Groups

Family fund, P.O. Box 50, York YO1 1VY.

The family fund is run by the Joseph Rowntree Memorial Trust. Objective to help families caring for the severely handicapped child under the age of 16 years. Write for application form if you should need help with laundry equipment, clothing, bedding, footwear, holiday for the whole family and so forth.

Designers, Manufacturers and Suppliers of Toys

John Adams Toys Ltd.,
Crazies Hill,
Wargrave, Berks.

E. J. Arnold & Son Ltd.,
Parkside Lane,
Dewsbury Road,
Leeds LS11 5TD.

Escor Toys Ltd.,
Groveley Road,
Christchurch,
Dorset.

Fisher-Price Toys,
P.O. Box 100,
Peterlee
Co. Durham SR8 2RF.

James Galt & Co. Ltd.,
Brookfield Road,
Cheadle,
Cheshire SK8 2PN.

Kiddicraft Ltd.,
Redlands Coulsdon,
Surrey CR3 2HR.

Susan Wynter Toys,
Toy Trumpet Workshops Ltd.,
Church Road,
Brighlingsea,
Essex.

INDEX

Acceptance, 12, 13
  of help, 15
  social, 16
'Adjustable Rolator Walker', 194
Adjustment, 13
Age and development, 1
Aggressiveness, 26
Anoraks, 109
Approval, 23
Associated reactions, 124, 260, 263
Ataxic child, co-ordination of movement, 239
Athetoid child, 56
  abnormal postures, 53
  bathing, 85
  body awareness, 217
  bouncing, 47
  carrying, 142
  chairs for, 159, 168, 170
  dressing, 91, 98, 101
  feeding, 123
  grasp, 255
  handling, 46
  movement, 34, 39, 40, 44
  prams, 152
  push-chair, 153
  reaching out, 213
  sitting balance, 158
  sitting position, 66, 71, 72
  throwing in air, 47
Attention, 208
  means of attracting, 28-9
  seeking at night, 74

'Baby Bouncers', 47
'Baby Buggy', 153
'Baby Bumper' pads, 74
'Baby Relax Toilette', 76
Baby-sitter, 16
Balance, 217, 219, 221, 273
Balance-board, 196
Ball, choice of, 233
  correct use of, 241
  play therapy, 297
  sitting and lying on, 246-8
  use in play, 256

Ball run, 254
Bath seats, 85, 161
Bathing, 82-9
  baby, 82
  equipment suppliers, 293
  importance of balance, 82
  independence in, 88
  older child, 84, 89
  use of false bottom, 87
Bathroom equipment, 89
Bavin, Jack, 12
'Bean Bag' chair, 70, 159
Bed, position of, 68
Behaviour, questionnaire, 283
  social, 22-4
Behavioural problems, 27
Bibs, 109
Body-manipulation, 27
Books, 295
  choice and use of, 138
Bottle-drinking, 118
Bouncing on the floor, 46
'Bouncing Cradle', 179, 228
Bowel control, 81
Brain, effects of damage to, 33
Brain cells, damaged, 203-4
Breathing, 135
Bricks, 233
Bridging, 39
'Buggy Major', 153
'Bunny-hopping', 45
'Busy-box', 234, 244

Car, without pedals, 199
Car seat, 'Star Rider', 162
Cardboard box, as chair, 166
  as play area, 166
Carrying, 139-50
  aids, 144
  athetoid child, 142
  'floppy' child, 144
  position, 139
  questionnaire, 278
  spastic child, 139-42
Chairs, 156-78

and tables, 175-8
basic requirements, 156
'Bean-Bag', 159
box-type, with tray, 164
cardboard box as, 166
corner seat, 172
cylinder, 167
foam shapes, 174
inflatable, 159
'Mountain', 169
packing cases, 174
proprietory types, 161-4, 168-76
roller, 168, 197
    with cut-out table, 177
round inflatable, 161
suppliers, 290
triangle, 168
triangle inflatable, 159
'T.V.' plastic and steel-framed, 163
see also Sitting
Chewing, 120
'Cheyne Walk Bar', 194
Clothes, choice of, 100
    choice of materials, 104
    for babies, 110
    suitable types of, 104-10
Coats, 109
Colour, learning about, 241
Communication, 211, 274
    difficulties in, 209
Community projects, 31
Concentration, 8, 237, 238
Confidence in learning, 202-3
'Cosco Go-Go' seat, 162
Cot, position of, 68
Creeping on tummy, 39
Criticism, 23, 26
Cutlery, building up handles, 293

Deafness, 7
Dental care, 128-30
Dentist, visits to, 130
Development, and age, 1
    cerebral palsied child, ix-xi
    intellectual, 18
    normal, ix, 2, 32, 51, 211
        dressing, 90
        early stages of, 266-74
        feeding, 111-12, 122-3
        play, 227, 238
        speech, 131
    optimal, 17
    social, 18
Disapproval, 23, 24
Discipline, 22
Doll's house, 234

Dresses, 105
Dressing, 5, 90-110
    athetoid child, 98, 101
    communication during, 96-7
    fastenings, 109
    hemiplegic child, 97, 99
    independence in, 90, 94-5, 206
    lying on side, 92
    physical difficulties, 99-100
    position, 91
    questionnaire, 282
    sitting on lap, 93
    spastic child, 98, 101, 103
Dribbling, 118
Drinking, 112, 121-2
    equipment suppliers, 292
    with polyester tube, 122

Education attainment, social behaviour rather than, 30
Effort, excessive, 7
Embarrassment, 14
Emotional needs, 14
Encouragement, 20, 23-4, 26, 208
Experiments, 231
Expression, forms of, 7
Eye-hand co-ordination, 212-13, 255-8, 260, 269
Eye-hand development, 273
Eye-hand regard, 267, 271

Family, effects on, 14, 16
Fastenings, 109
Father, attitude of, 14
    role of, 19
Feeding, 8, 9, 20, 21, 111-30
    athetoid child, 123
    bottle-drinking, 118
    chewing, 120
    controlling mouth functioning, 117
    drinking, 112, 121-2, 292
    equipment suppliers, 292
    from spoon, 118
    gadgets, 127
    hemiplegic child, 124
    independence in, 122
    link with speech patterns, 128
    normal development, 111-12, 122-3
    positions, 113
    problems of, 26, 112
    questionnaire, 276
    spastic diplegic child, 123
    spastic quadruplegic child, 123
Fighting, 26
Financial assistance, 10
Fire hazards, 10-11

Foam, fire hazard, 10-11
Foam shapes as chairs, 174
Food, avoidance of sugary, 129
Frustration, 7, 237
Functional activities, handling in, 5
Future, worrying about, 21-2

'Gaiter' splint, 188
Games, 19, 27, 232, 235
Garage, 244
Gardner, Mary, 200
Gestures, 137
Glossary, 287
Gloves, 109
Grasp, 211-25, 255, 269
    and movement, 221
    stages in development of, 218, 220
Groin straps, in push-chair, 153
Guilt, 13
Gums, brushing, 130

Hammock, 72, 179, 228
Hand-biting, 29
Hand regard, 268
Handling, basic principles of, 51-67
    bouncing on floor, 46
    in functional activities, 5
    methods not recommended, 45-50
    pulling up to sitting from lying on back, 46
    swinging in air, 47
    throwing in air, 47
Hands, and eyes, co-ordination between, 212-13, 255-8, 260, 269
    development of, 211
    encouraging use of, 248-9
    helping in use of, 229
    of spastic child, 59
Hats, 109
Head-banging, 29, 74
Head control, 51, 54-5, 96, 144, 151, 165, 182, 266, 267, 271
Hearing and hearing defects, 7, 133, 269, 271
Help, acceptance of, 15
    seeking additional, 31
Hemiplegic child, 261
    abnormal postures, 53
    associated reactions, 260, 263
    dressing, 97, 99
    feeding, 124
    movement, 35
    play, 231, 262, 264, 265
High-chair, 156
Hoops, 195
Hospital, going into, 9
Hypersensitivity, 118

Imitation, 258
    learning by, 202
Independence, 10, 17, 89, 211
    in dressing, 90, 94-5, 206
    in feeding, 122
    in washing and bathing, 88
    need to encourage, 6, 206
Intellectual development, 18
Intelligence, measurement of, 203
Intelligence tests, 204-5
Interview with therapist, 3
IQ, 204, 205

Jaw control, 117, 118, 120, 165
Jerseys, 105
Jig-saw puzzle, 240

Key-points, 51, 52
Kneeling, 253

Lavatory, aids to use of, 81
Learning, basic mental and physical equipment for, 203
    basic perception, 245
    handicapped child, 202
    need for encouragement in, 206-7
    normal child, 201-2
    process of, 18
    special difficulties, 207
    stimulation in, 206, 209-10
    through play, 226
Legs, parting, 58
Lifting, spastic child, 142
Listening, 8
Lying on stomach, moving away from, 34

Magnetic boards, 240
Magnifying glass, 235
Manipulation, 211-25, 271, 273
    and speech, 214
    and vision, 271, 272
Matchbox furniture, 243
Materials, 104
Mealtimes, 8
Mini-prone board, 188
Mobility, aids to, 191-9
Moro reaction, 82-3
Mother, as teacher, 18
    attitude of, 14
    communication with, 211
    contact with, 18
Motor patterns, 269
'Mountain' chair, 169
Mouth, open, 118, 135-6
Movement, 32-50
    abnormal, to be discouraged, 45

abnormal patterns of, 53
abnormally performed, 39-45
and eye-hand control, 257-8
and grasp, 221
and play, 232
athetoid child, 34, 39, 40, 44
basic differences between normal and abnormal sequences of, 33-5
bridging, 39
'bunny-hopping', 45
creeping on tummy, 39
from lying on stomach, 34
hemiplegic child, 35
improving quality of, 35
pushing backwards on floor, 39
questionnaire, 279
resistance to, 51
rolling, 34
sitting up from lying on back, 33
spastic child, 39, 44
spastic diplegic child, 34, 40
standing and taking a step, 44
Mueller, Helen, 111, 131
Muscle tone, changes of, 51
Muscles, 32
Music, 234

Nappy liners, 81
National Society for Mentally Handicapped Children, 13
Negativism, 21, 27
Nightdresses, 104
Notebook, 6

Obstacle course, 225, 232
Obstinacy, 24-6
Operation, preparation for, 9
Oral therapy, 212
Overalls, 109, 124
Over-attachment, 29-30
Over-protection, 29-30

Packing cases as chairs, 174
Pants, 104
Parent-child relationship, 29, 138
  changing, 17
  establishing, 16
Parents, attitude of, 14
  co-operation of, 1, 3
  development, 17, 24
  distress of, 12, 22
  expectations of, 203
  problems of, 12-31
  relationship with experts, 200
  task facing, 22

Personal interaction in speech development, 138
Pëto chair, 176
Pillows, 74
Play, 27, 226-65
  and movement, 232
  cerebral palsied child, 227
    able to balance and to move, 232
  first steps in, 228
  helping in, 237-8
  hemiplegic child, 262, 264, 265
  importance of, 19
  in foam case, 252
  interference by parent, 237
  learning through, 226
  moderately affected child, 231
  normal child, 227
  position, 228, 242, 251, 253
  questionnaire, 284
  severely handicapped or very young cerebral palsied child, 227
  two to three-year-old cerebral palsied child, 239
  two-year-old normal child, 238
Play area, cardboard box as, 166
Pleasure, 19
Plunger, 237
Posting box, 236
Postures, abnormal, 53
Pot, type and position of, 76
Potty chair, 76
Prams, 151-2
Prone boards, 185, 297
Psychologist, role of, 200-10
Pulling up to sitting from lying on back, 46
Push-chairs, 152-5
  suppliers, 290
Pushing backwards on floor, 39
Pyjamas, 104

Questionnaire, 275-86
  use of, 2
Quoit rings, 195

Reaching out, 213, 216, 270
Rebellion, 21
Records, 296
Reflex walking, 44
Rejection, 12
Repetition, 6
Resistance to movement, 51
Response, waiting for, 19-20
Responsibility, 31
Restlessness, 74
Riding, 10
Roller, 253

correct use of, 241
placing child over, 62
'Roller Chair', 168, 197
   with cut-out table, 177
Rolling, 34, 266, 269, 271
Rotation, 34, 257, 269, 271

'Saddle Seat Engine', 168, 197
'Safa' bath seat, 86, 161
Scrap book, 234
Screaming, 28, 29
Self-control, 23, 25
Self-help, encouragement of, 20
Sensory experience, 202
Sensory input, 136
Sensory-motor involvement, 135
Sensory-motor preparation, 138
Separation-anxiety, 30
Shame, 14
Shape, visual concept of, 241
Shape differentiation and recognition, 239
Shirts, 105
Shoes, 106-8
   odd, 107
   protection, 107
   suppliers, 294
Sitting, 63, 64, 65, 113-14, 178, 182, 250, 268
   athetoid child, 66, 158
   spastic child, 66
   see also Chairs
Sitting up from lying on back, 33
Sleep and sleeping, 68-74
   equipment suppliers, 294
   questionnaire, 281
Sleeplessness, 74
Sleeves, 105
Smacking, 26
Social acceptance, 16
Social behaviour, 22-4
   rather than educational attainment, 30
Social contact, 28, 30
Social development, 18
Social isolation, 14
Social needs, 14
Social services, 10
Socks, 105
Spastic child, x, 5, 56, 57, 63
   abnormal postures, 53
   bathing, 85
   bouncing, 47
   carrying, 139-42
   dressing, 91, 98, 101, 103
   hand of, 59
   lifting, 142
   movement, 39, 44
   prams, 152

reaching out, 213, 216
sitting positions, 66
sleeping position, 71
standing position, 67
throwing in air, 47
Spastic diplegic child, chairs, 168
   feeding, 123
   handling, 46
   mobility aid, 192
   movement, 34, 40
Spastic hemiplegic child, chair for, 161
Spastic quadruplegic child, feeding, 123
Spastics Society, 13, 107
Speech, 131-8, 269, 271, 272, 274
   and manipulation, 214
   and motor performance, 209
   common problems of, 135
   defects, 7-9
   development, 8, 19, 133
      gestures in, 137
      in normal child, 131
      personal interaction in, 138
      sensory input in, 136
   feeding patterns link with, 128
   playing with, 137
   preparation for, 133
   questionnaire, 277
   special problems of, 132
Spider Walker, 198
Standing, 254
   aid to, 188
   and taking a step, 44
   spastic child, 67
'Star Rider' car seat, 162
Steerable Walker, 198
Stimulation in learning, 206, 209-10
Sucking-swallowing reflex, 111, 117
'Suzy Inflatable Chair', 85
Swallowing, 114
Swimming, 10
Swinging in air, 47
Symmetry, 212

Tables and chairs, 175-8
Tactile experiences, 213
Tactile perception, 252
Tantrums, 24-6
Teaching, guiding principles of, 20
   mother's role in, 18
Teeth, care of, 128-30
   cleaning, 128-9
Tenseness, 7
Therapist, discussions with, 4-5
   interview with, 3
Throwing in air, 47
Tights, 105

Toes, straightening, 58
Toilet equipment suppliers, 293
Toilet seats, 79
Toilet training, 27, 75-81
    general points to bear in mind, 81
    questionnaire, 281
Toothbrush, electric, 129
Toy frame, 175, 235
Toy libraries, 10, 233
Toys, 19, 24
    bath, 84
    choice of, 233
    designers, manufacturers and suppliers, 298
Treatment, aim of, 3
    approach to, 4
    early, 3
    importance of, 3
    planning, 3

Tricycle, 197, 198, 199
Trousers, 106
Tunnel, 74

Vests, 104
Vision, and eye-hand co-ordination, 269
    and eye-hand regard, 267
    and manipulation, 271, 272
    and motor performance, 208
Visual defects, 7
Visual perception, handicaps, 207

Walking, aids, 193-6
    reflex, 44
Washing, independence in, 88
    questionnaire, 280
Wedges, 182, 196, 252, 297
Wellingtons, 108
Worry, 22